PRELUDE TO CHANGE

Struggling to Survive With Chronic Kidney Failure

BY

George Van Giesen, Jr. M.D.

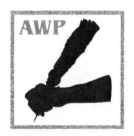

The Ardent Writer Press
Brownsboro, Alabama

GEORGE VAN GIESEN, JR. M.D.

Struggling to Survive

PRELUDE TO CHANGE

with Chronic Kidney Failure

An Ardent Writer Press Book
Brownsboro, Alabama

Photos are from the author or from multiple public domain and credited sources, including Wikipedia and Pixabay.com. One photo is courtesy of Nancy Spaeth, initiated with the assistance of Dr. Neil Turner, University of Edinburgh (UK), Professor of Nephrology, Queen's Medical Research Institute (CIR). Line art images are composites created by The Ardent Writer Press using photoshop techniques.

ISBN 978-1-938667-65-7 (pbk); 978-1-938667-49-7 (hbk)

Library of Congress Control Number: 2016962904
Library of Congress subject headings:
- Chronic renal failure.
- Chronic renal failure--History.
- Chronic renal failure--Patients--Care
- Chronic renal failure--Psychological aspects.
- Chronic renal failure--Treatment--United States--Case studies.

First Edition

PREFACE

LESLIE, PLEASE DON'T CRY?

The dialysis is finished.
She breaths with lesser force.
The excess fluid removed,
A change effected in her course.
Kidneys scarred beyond repair.
A transient recourse.
Still, the nausea has abated.
The frost all gone away.
Her creatinine is down again.
It certainly won't stay.
Only a matter of time—there's little
more to say ...

Except:
The diet is unpalatable.
She balks at every meal.
If only she'd eat all of it—there's a good
chance she'd feel
better in a week or so.
But twenty grams of protein, what a sorry deal.

And:
Before the frost reappeared,
We asked about her kin.
Brothers, sisters, mom, dad?

We'd like to talk to them.
"Adopted at age three," she said.
"Nineteen years ago."
"I never knew my ma or pa."

So:
"Transplantation's out for now,"
says Dr. Richard Crowe.

And:
The fistula's thrombosed.
It worked for seven days
Crowe's a bit upset..
"It passed the crucial phase,"

He said.
"These vessels are much too small.
We'll give it another try.
This time a larger vein.
Take it from the thigh — and hope."

But now:
The miseries have returned.
The nausea and the heaves.
She's depressed — who wouldn't be?
Are there no reprieves?

Hope:
Get out the tray.
Yes, the one we used before.
Now prep her belly gently.
That old wound's still sore.
Leslie, please don't cry.

George Van Giesen, Jr. M.D.
April 6, 1970

ACKNOWLEDGMENTS

Though, to protect their identity, this memoir alters the names of some of the patients and other persons and places described herein, the stories are real. I respect and honor the memories of my patients' courage in their struggle to survive in a time of little opportunity and much uncertainty. Their stories need telling.

There is no way I could have finished writing this book without the support of many people. I start with my wife, Sylvia. She has provided me with both emotional support and editorial skills. She has put up with my obsessive traits and labored long with me when I couldn't find just the right words to express myself. Her instructions to say what I want to say in as simple and direct a manner as possible have made passages in this book much clearer. Where there are obfuscations, they are mine alone.

Thanks go to Janet Holt., my first dialysis technician, Jeannie Carter Reeves, my first dialysis nurse, and to Patricia McKenney. my first dialysis secretary, for jogging my memory of events that occurred. in some instances, half a century ago.

Thanks to Harry Sherman, M.D. and Hy Sussman, MD. for reading early drafts and offering encouragement, recollections, and suggestions.

My daughter, Diane Van Giesen, read all my drafts. I rely on her knowledge of books and publishing to guide me in recording my memories on paper. I deeply appreciate her.

Gail Van Giesen was essential in clarifying many of my recollections of how and when things happened. She was an integral part of the tale. Many thanks.

I'm indebted to Wanda McBride and Alice Howell for allowing me to better understand the stresses and coping mechanisms of family members of patients with chronic renal failure.

I have many people to thank for spending hours of their lives helping me understand how to make my computer work properly. I received, and appreciate, guidance from my son, Eddie, and from my grandchildren, Ian Van Giesen, Cedric Van Giesen, Olivia Barrett, Hale Barrett, and Ezra Barrett. And special thanks go to Isabella Van Giesen and her mother, Viviane Van Giesen, who saved drafts of my early papers,. when I thought them lost.

My girls, Jennifer Best, Jessica Fasci, and Michelle Bennett read my first drafts and were always available to offer advice/suggestions and to work me through many computer challenges. And Nicholas Herring was also ready to help when my computer failed. I thank all of them.

Appreciation to Dave Bennett, without whose aid I would never have been able to finish this book on my own Mac.

I want to thank Diane Cantor, author of The Poisoned Table, for her suggestions and encouragement in seeking publication.

I thank Barbara Newborg, M.D. for sending me a copy of the Scientific Publications of Walter Kempner, M.D. along with her book, Walter Kempner and the Rice Diet.

I'm appreciative of Steve Gierhart's decision to publish *Prelude to Change*, and for his patience with my frequent desire to add/or change passages, and for his skill in ushering the book forward.

I have a much better understanding of what to say and how to say it because of Doyle Duke's skill as an editor. Thank you.

Many, many thanks to my nurses and technicians for their dedication to patient care.

CONTENTS

PREFACE

ACKNOWLEDGMENTS

CONTENTS

CHAPTER 1

*On October 30, 1972 President Richard Nixon signed **HR 1 (Public Law 92-603)** with welfare reform and a revision and extension of Medicare and Medicaid provisions as its chief elements. A brief attachment to this bill (**Section 2991**) extended Medicare coverage, for the first time, to patients with a specific disease. The resultant Medicare End Stage Renal Disease Program (ESRD) was implemented July 1, 1973. Now, Medicare covers over 90% of patients with chronic kidney failure.*

"The state inspectors are here," Janet Holt, my office manager, announced as she knocked on my door.

My office was across from Doctors Hospital in West Richmond County. I had finished making morning rounds at the new Augusta Dialysis Center adjoining the office and was sitting at my desk.

"Come in," I said, leaning back in my chair.

Janet, in her early forties, was an attractive blonde-haired woman with a sweet smile. She had worked for me, off and on, since I started practice, eleven years ago. Although not formerly trained as a nurse, after working in the Nephrology Department at the Medical College of Georgia (MCG) and in my dialysis clinic across the street, she had extensive experience in the frontline of nursing.

"It's about time they're here," I said. We had been dialyzing under the new Medicare regulations for six months, waiting to receive our Certificate of Compliance. I wondered if we should meet them at the Center now, or wait until they finished their inspection. "We're ready for them, aren't we?"

"Dr. George, I don't think it's a question of us being ready ... but are they ready for us?"

"The inspectors?"

"Yes, the inspectors. They've never inspected a dialysis facility. In fact, they've never been in, or seen, one. They're Nursing Home inspectors, and we're the first Dialysis Center in this part of the state they've chosen to inspect."

"You mean we're to be inspected by nursing home inspectors to determine if we're in compliance for running a dialysis center?" I said incredulously.

"Right, but maybe we can help."

"Really? How?"

"Well, before I left the Center, I was sitting in my office, just watching them. They huddled by the front door, looking around the building — but mostly looking at each other — like maybe they were thinking, who or what should we inspect first? I think we could give them some ideas as to what we think they might, or should, be looking for to determine if a dialysis facility is safe enough to pass inspection."

"I suppose we could offer to give them an *inservice* of sorts." I sat up in my chair and considered the situation in its absurdity.

Ten minutes later, all three of the Dialysis Center Inspectors gathered in my office with Janet and me. They introduced themselves as Terri, Jane, and Horace. Horace offered that they had a combined 35 years of inspecting Nursing Homes for the State of Georgia.

Horace, thin, balding, probably in his early fifties, seemed to be in charge. He explained, "The State gave us guidelines and brochures explaining what a dialysis center does, so we do have some general idea of its functioning. However, when we were actually *in* your center and saw all those patients, sitting in recliners next to the dialysis machines, with tubes in their arms, and blood flowing through the tubes, we were a bit overwhelmed. We didn't know where to start."

I looked at the clock on my desk. In another 30 minutes my first morning patients would begin arriving. I told them Janet and I would do our best to point out some specific issues we felt were important for the proper and safe functioning of a dialysis center. They whipped out their yellow legal pads and began taking notes.

We explained the basic functioning of dialysis: diverting blood from a patient, running it through a dialyzer submerged in a 'dialyzing' solution, transferring toxic products from the blood, through the dialyzer membrane, into the dialyzing fluid; thereby cleansing the blood and returning it to the patient. We emphasized the sterile techniques and safety measures that were necessary for successful dialysis and pointed out the various monitoring devices.

Janet explained the importance of having adequate numbers of well-trained nurses and technicians in attendance at all times. She pointed out that we had ten dialysis stations and were dialyzing all patients for six hours, one group Monday, Wednesday, and Friday and another group Tuesday, Thursday, and Saturday. She explained the ratios of nurses/technicians to patients — one to two — that we insisted on having in our center. The inspectors busily jotted down as much of what we told them as they could, trying to take in all of the new information. They asked few questions.

Horace and his team left my office and returned to the Dialysis Center to "inspect." Three hours later, as I was seeing my last morning patient, Janet stopped me in the hall. "The inspectors have finished." She hesitated a moment, then a broad smile flashed across her face. "We passed. Now, we're an official part of the End Stage Renal Disease (ESRD) network! They said that they wanted to express their appreciation to us for our help, and wished us all the best; and that they would probably see us again next year." She added that they drove off in separate cars, probably relieved to have successfully inspected their first dialysis center.

"*How's that for bureaucratic efficiency,*" I thought to myself, as I walked back to the dialysis center. The patients had settled into their routine of enduring the long hours of dialysis. All were in La-Z-Boy recliners. Some were watching their chair side televisions, others reading their magazines or books, and others just sleeping. Dialyzing patients with chronic kidney failure had not always been so orderly and efficient.

CHAPTER 2

THE EARLY YEARS

*First proposed by President Kennedy in 1963, **The Civil Rights Act, HR 7152, Public law 88-352,** was signed by President Johnson July 2, 1964. Among its many provisions, racial discrimination in any accommodations engaged in interstate commerce was prohibited.*

In early July 1963, I returned to Augusta to begin my new life in the private practice of medicine. I had spent the last two years in Dallas, at the University of Texas Southwestern Medical School, completing a Fellowship in Metabolism/ Renal Medicine under Donald W. Seldin, M.D.

At that time, there were no privately practicing physicians in Augusta who limited their practice to medical — non-surgical — diseases of the kidney. The term Nephrology, describing those physicians' specialty, was not one widely recognized outside of academic medicine. Urology referred to physicians trained in surgical aspects of kidney disease. On my prescription pads and on my office sign, I referred to myself as practicing Internal Medicine/Renal Disease.

John Phinizy, with whom I had been in residency training at the Medical College of Georgia (MCG) in Augusta, had invited me to join him in practice when I finished my fellowship training. John had been in General Practice for several years in Lincolnton, a small town an hour's drive from Augusta. He had returned to his hometown, Augusta, and MCG, to begin a Residency in Internal Medicine.

One day, after we had made morning hospital rounds and were taking a coffee break, John explained that there were a number of reasons for his leaving Lincolnton. He had no one he could count on regularly with whom to share calls. He found he had little time for himself. "Lots of time," he said, "I'd come home from working in my office all day and find three or four patients sitting on my front porch — rocking and chatting with each other, waiting for me. There was no hospital in the county and, therefore, no emergency room. I ended up treating too many patients for serious injuries and illnesses at home — theirs or mine — when they should have been in the hospital."

"I guess some of the things that gave me real pause," he continued, "as to whether or not this was the life I really wanted to be living, was when I began to think and talk in lay terms about my patients' illnesses. I remember telling one patient 'you've got a bad case of the high blood' and another, 'I'm worried that you may have the bad blood.' I felt I needed more contact with medical professionals, at least some of the time, instead of always talking just with my patients."

John was in his mid-thirties, short, with thinning red hair and pale skin. He had been my resident physician while I was an intern. John was an excellent doctor. He could evaluate a patient's condition in short order, sorting out the relevant facts from the irrelevant ones, coming quickly to a working diagnosis. When it came to formulating lab, x ray studies, and other diagnostics pursuant to a final diagnosis and treatment plan, he was very efficient. He didn't suffer fools, but he was understanding, compassionate, and his patients loved him. I felt fortunate to be his associate.

John's office was small. It was located in a medical office complex adjacent to the old University Hospital, a facility long used both for teaching medical students from the Medical College of Georgia and for doctors in private practice in the

Augusta area. In fact, University Hospital was the primary teaching hospital for the Medical College of Georgia until the Eugene Talmadge Memorial Hospital (ETMH) was completed in 1954. Medical students and residents still rotated through University and most of the physicians in our medical complex. John and I, along with many others in our complex, were on the Clinical Facility of the Medical College.

Because of limited space in the office, John and I worked out a plan so we both wouldn't be there at the same time. I would see patients when he was making rounds in the hospital, and vice-versa. His secretary, Dorothy Bohler, answered the phone and made appointments for both of us. She also assisted us in the exam rooms, continued to help me in the office, and transcribed my dictation. This was a tremendous boon for me because I had practically no savings at that time. I have always felt deeply indebted to John and Dorothy, for their generosity in helping me make the transition from training, to private practice.

After about six months, I felt successful enough to hire my own secretary. During the fall and into the winter, as my practice increased, it became obvious that we needed a larger office. John contacted a local builder, Jerry Holden, who had done some add-on work to his home. After discussions, we contracted with Jerry to construct an office for us, to our specifications, on a property Jerry owned on Central Ave, between University and St. Joseph hospitals.

Jerry knew nothing about building doctors' offices. His building experiences were mainly with convenience stores. But thinking we knew exactly what we wanted in the way of an office, we told him that we would design it ourselves, without the assistance of an architect.

THE SIXTIES were times of great social changes in this country and especially in the South. Augusta harbored many unreconstructed segregationists. Roy Harris, a state senator for many years, published a rabid, segregationist newspaper. He was one of those politicians who had no intention of allowing the Federal government, or any government, to change his entrenched way of behavior and thinking. He was a strict believer in Alabama Governor Wallace's firmly held conviction of "segregation now, segregation tomorrow, and segregation forever." These were unsettled times.

The Civil Rights Act of 1964 outlawed segregation in public places that engaged in interstate commerce. John and I were unsure as to how this legislation would affect physicians in private practice. The regulations were not clear about this issue. In reviewing the statute, we found that private medical offices were not specifically mentioned in Title II, section 201, the section listing establishments that must be "in compliance."

Both John and I had lived, practically our entire lives, in segregated environments, which we had come to accept as "the norm." There were no "black" students in my classes in undergraduate school at Emory University, in Atlanta, and none in my classes at the Medical College of Georgia, in Augusta. This is not to say that medical students in the South didn't come in close contact with African Americans. Probably, half the patients we saw as medical students "on the wards," and later during internship, residency, and fellowship training were of African descent. Moreover, we took histories and performed physicals on them in the same manner as we did on all our patients—complete in every sense of the word.

Looking back on those days, from the perspective of today, it's difficult to understand why I, along with many other white southerners, never seriously considered that our segregated way of life ever needed to change. Until the civil rights protests of the late fifties and the early sixties, I had not considered the effect of segregation on the lives of African Americans in the South. I was not so naive to think that all was right in the black communities of the South—or the North, for that matter. It was more like, "out of sight out of mind."

I knew that "black schools" were inferior to "white schools." I didn't know how inferior. I knew that the teachers in black schools were not as well qualified as teachers in white schools. I didn't know how poorly qualified. I knew that living conditions of African Americans were not up to the standards of most Caucasians, but I rarely thought about this. After all, I rarely visited those sections of town.

However, I didn't think of myself as being of the same breed as many of those unreconstructed Southern politicians. Both John and I treated our African American patients with the same degree of consideration and concern for their illnesses as we did for our Caucasian patients. The only difference was we expected them to use separate waiting rooms in our offices and in our hospitals. When they were admitted to the hospital, they were assigned rooms on a separate floor from Caucasian patients.

At that time, a few Southern states had passed laws specifically requiring segregation in public hospitals. While Georgia laws only required segregation for mental patients, University Hospital had its own regulations requiring segregation on the treatment floors as well as in waiting rooms. The Barrett wing was for Caucasian patients and the Lamar wing for African Americans.

Were we naive to think that these African American patients wanted to be segregated? Probably. Perhaps, some did prefer separation from Caucasians, whose presence alone disturbed them. But others, surely, resented this overt discrimination.

IN THE SOUTH, where I grew up, this was "just the way it is." It had been like this for decades and decades. Also, It was the way the Federal Government deemed it should be. For almost 60 years, from 1896, when the Supreme Court issued its decision in Plessy v. Ferguson, until 1954, when Chief Justice Earl Warren's Court delivered its unanimous ruling, (Brown v. Board of Education), banning the prior interpretation of constitutional law, "separate but equal" was the law of the land.

In 1955, the Warren Court issued another decision, (Brown II) affirming its earlier action, and calling for states to desegregate "with deliberate speed." However, it wasn't until almost a decade later, with the Civil Rights Act of 1964, that it became obvious, to even stanch Southern segregationists, that the fight to maintain the status quo was nearing an end.

The Civil Rights Act of 1964 certainly was the catalyst that stimulated my thinking about the integration movement, and the conditions under which African Americans had been living since their ancestors were freed from slavery a century earlier. And probably, if not for the fact that this bill impacted directly on our livelihood, John and I might have been less inclined to think about the civil rights movement the way we did.

When I joined John in practice, at least half of his patients were African American. Months later, our practices were still about equally divided between Caucasians and African Americans. When building our new offices, we came to the decision that it would be best to desegregate. Finally, we had come to realize that the old order of segregation, with "separate but equal" everything, was no longer legally acceptable.

For decades, there had been "Colored" waiting rooms, "Colored" water fountains, and "Colored" restrooms in all public accommodations through the South. When I joined John, all of these segregated areas were integral parts of his office — as in most other Augusta medical offices. We were in a dilemma as to how to incorporate features of the new order into the design and construction of our new facility. We were concerned that few white Augustans were ready to accept total integration — certainly not in close social environments. Yet, we knew that "separate but equal" facilities were going to be difficult to defend. Moreover, I think both of us had developed a more liberal approach to racial issues.

So, we designed one main waiting room, and on the other side of the entrance hallway, another "overflow" waiting room of slightly smaller size. We hoped our African American patients would understand that this was their waiting room.

Although it was not quite as large as the main waiting room, we did not intend it to be inferior in design and function to the other waiting room. Each room had its own water fountain and restroom. No signs were posted indicating a distinction. For the next several years, our African American patients continued to segregate themselves. They moved to this alternate waiting room without ever being so directed. I admit I was surprised that none ever said a word to us, or our staff, about this voluntary way of maintaining a separation of the races. In retrospect, I suspect they may have been afraid of complaining—maybe fearing they wouldn't be seen or treated if they voiced discontent. I don't know.

Over the next two years, we came to realize that our architectural design wasn't working. Moreover, we found that, in fact, it was inferior in both function and design. The corridor leading to the overflow waiting room was too narrow to accommodate wheelchairs. It was too narrow for some of our obese patients, who found that the only way to their waiting area was to turn sidewise and waddle through.

Later, we thought it was time to correct the gross inefficiencies of design in our office building and to be, not only politically, but also morally, ethically, and socially correct. We contracted with a different builder and began our reconstruction.

We eliminated the two waiting rooms by tearing down the wall between them, creating one large reception area. The extra restroom was redesigned for my personal use only—instead of John and I sharing the one we had before. Now, we had only one water fountain and one restroom for all our patients. Again, no patients complained about any of the changes we had made. Integration evolved in our professional lives without disturbances.

CHAPTER 3

RITA KIMBLE

Life is short, and Art long; the crisis fleeting; experience perilous, and decision difficult. **Aphorisms by Hippocrates circa 400 B.C.E.** *Translated from the Greek by Francis Adams.*

I was uncertain as to what type of medical practice I would have when I began my association with John. His was a big, general medical practice, much akin to the one he had in Lincolnton. Except now, he didn't see children, pregnant women, or trauma patients. I knew he would be sending me some of his patients, because his practice had grown considerably since he had been back in Augusta.

I was able to supplement my income by managing the University Hospital Outpatient Medicine Clinic. I was responsible for overseeing medical students who rotated through the clinic, which accepted indigent patients from Richmond County – and beyond. Dorothy Peterson and Melba Fair, both RNs, managed all nursing aspects of the clinic in a very personable and professional manner. They guided patients through their clinic visits with kindness, compassion, and skill. Many patients, with less serious illnesses, looked forward to their clinic visits. They enjoyed the socialization with other patients, the medical students, and the nurses, who treated them all with respect.

In late summer of 1964, Rita Kimble, a 45-year-old mother of four, was referred to me by Dr. Donald Mixon, who had both an Ob/Gyn and General Practice in South Augusta. Dr. Mixon had attended all of Mrs. Kimble's six pregnancies, two of which had resulted in miscarriages.

On the phone, Dr. Mixon told me, "During the third trimester of her last pregnancy, five years ago, Mrs. Kimble had very high blood pressures, along with extensive swelling of both legs. She made it safely through delivery, with a viable birth of a healthy son. Then, I lost track of her. She showed up in my office two days ago—five years after her last delivery. She had moved to Floyd County and told me she hadn't been seeing anyone about her medical condition. Her husband had been in an accident and had been out of work for several years. She decided to come back to see me because she hadn't been feeling well for the last two to three months. She has no appetite, and is nauseated constantly. I obtained blood work, which I'll have her bring. BUN (Blood Urea Nitrogen) is 140, Creatinine 9, and Hemoglobin (Hgb) 7. Can you work her in soon?"

I told him that I could see Mrs. Kimble the next afternoon. "Ask her to come in around two."

Mrs. Kimble showed up promptly the next day. She introduced me to her neighbor, Helen, who drove the two of them to Augusta in Helen's '59 Ford pickup.

Mrs. Kimble was a small woman and looked somewhat older than her years. There was puffiness about her face. She wore her gray-streaked hair in a bun. Her makeup failed to conceal her pallid complexion. She said she was nauseous most of the time and had no desire for food.

I found no past history of kidney problems or other significant diseases or conditions. She mentioned that she had two older sisters who were being treated for "high blood."

On examination, she weighed 140 pounds and was 5' 2" in height. Her blood pressure (BP) was 220/120. Her mucous membranes were extremely pale and there were excoriations over her arms and legs, the result of scratching. Her eye grounds showed evidence of long standing hypertension; but there were no hemorrhages, exudates, or swelling of the optic discs.

"Doc," she said matter of factually, "I know I shouldn't be scratchin' all the time, but I can't seem to find anything 'cept scratchin' that helps, and it don't help all that much. And I know my pressure's up. I can always tell by the way my head throbs."

The remainder of my exam revealed swelling of her legs up to the thighs. Sitting upright, her neck veins were full. Her heart was greatly enlarged and beating at a rate of 110 per minute. There were fine to medium rales in both lung bases.

In my office, I examined Mrs. Kimble's spun urine sediment under the microscope. There was a large number of casts — a reflection of kidney damage. The urine gave a 2+ reaction for protein. I suspected that her kidney dysfunction was nephrosclerosis, related to her long-standing hypertension.

When I finished my evaluation, I sat down with her in my office. There were no family members with her. She explained that Luke, her oldest child, was unable to get off work today, and that her husband was still unable to drive. "He's at home mindin' the young' uns."

"Mrs. Kimble," I began, "like Dr. Mixon told you, the kidneys are the problem. Just how seriously damaged, I can't say for sure at this time. But we'll be able to determine their degree of injury shortly. It's best that we admit you to the hospital for further tests."

"Well, I was suspectin' as much, Doc. Doc Mixon told me you would probably want to have me admitted. I brought my suitcase with me. I told Herbert, my husband, not to 'spect me back tonight. I'm feelin' so bad I'm willin' to try anythin' to git better."

"I'll have Janet make arrangements for you to be admitted to University tonight — if there is a bed," I said.

Admitting a patient to the hospital in those days wasn't as complicated as it is today. Layers of bureaucracy were not as thick as they are now. This was before Medicaid, or at least

Medicaid in Georgia, had begun to function fully. Individual counties were responsible for reimbursing hospitals for the care of their indigent patients. Some of the counties near Richmond were not always prompt in taking financial responsibility for their indigent citizens sent to our county hospitals. However, they usually admitted the patient if the doctor explained to the admission office that it was an emergency, and if beds were available. Subsequent admissions of the same indigent, out of county patient, were often more difficult to arrange — especially if the bill for the initial hospitalization had not been finalized.

On rounds that evening, I ordered more blood work, medications for nausea, and placed Mrs. Kimble on a limited salt, low potassium diet. X-rays showed the outlines of two moderately shrunken kidneys. She had no evidence of any condition that might be obstructing the flow of urine. Further blood results showed that her serum electrolytes were deranged, that she was acidotic, along with low blood calcium and high blood phosphorus levels. These findings, along with creatinine clearances averaging 6 ml/min, reflected severely compromised kidney function. She remained nauseated and was able to eat little of the food on her plate. Rita Kimble was uremic (a condition in which failing kidneys are unable to eliminate toxins from the body) and in an advanced stage of chronic progressive kidney failure.

CHAPTER 4

BRIGHTS DISEASE

"I have never yet examined the body of a patient dying with dropsy, attended with coagulable urine, in whom some obvious derangement was not discovered in the kidneys." **Bright, Richard, Reports of Medical cases selected with a view of Illustrating the Symptoms and Cure of diseases by Reference to Morbid Anatomy, London, Longman, 1827, Vol 1, p. 1.**
Quoted from Classical Descriptions of Disease, Ralph H. Major, third Edition, August 1959 Charles Thomas, Publisher.

In the early 19th century, chronic kidney failure was not recognized as a specific illness. Kidney disease was often accompanied by dropsy, a condition in which large amounts of fluid accumulate throughout the body. But dropsy also was frequently a major feature of both heart failure and liver failure. For hundreds of years, dropsy was considered a disease in itself.

Richard Bright, working in Guys Hospital, London in the early 1800s, is considered to be the first to recognize the clinical syndrome of dropsy, coagulable urine (an indication of albumin in the urine), and damaged kidneys confirmed at autopsy. In 1827 and again in 1831, Bright published his findings in *Reports of Medical Cases*.

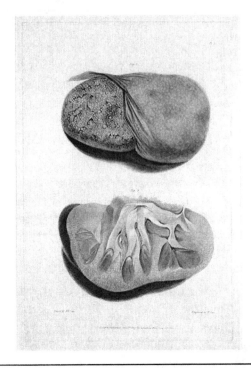

*Illustration of a diseased kidney from Richard Bright's Reports
of Medical Cases, Longman, London (1827–1831)*

Until the early 1960s, chronic renal failure, almost universally, was treated conservatively. By the 1950s, major medical textbooks, and textbooks of kidney diseases, referred to hemodialysis (artificial kidney), and peritoneal dialysis, as having been shown to be effective in reversing the manifestations of kidney failure. However, these procedures were ordinarily reserved for patients with acute renal failure, not patients with chronic kidney failure. These guidelines were to change rapidly over the next decade.

The rice diet of Walter Kempner, M.D. at Duke, also was effective in treating chronic kidney disease, as well as severe hypertension and cardiac disease, but never gained mainstream acceptance. I will discuss this later.

Often, in the early 1960s, chronic renal disease (CRD) was referred to as chronic Bright's disease. Although many different diseases were known to cause chronic progressive kidney failure, the late clinical and pathophysiologic manifestations of the chronically failing kidneys, and the progressively "downhill" course of the patients were basically the same. The generally accepted management of patients with chronic kidney failure until the late 1950s was palliative. In the early 1960s, treatment was still very conservative. Its objective was to correct the numerous bodily derangements and symptoms associated with the kidney's inability to maintain homeostasis. The therapeutic aims were to control blood pressure, regulate fluid intake, correct blood electrolyte disorders, insure proper nutrition, and mitigate as many of the other manifestations of the failing kidneys as possible. The Medical College of Georgia had an artificial kidney. It was used for acute, not chronic, kidney failure.

In the early 1960s, Dr. Belding Scribner's group in Seattle, Dr. John Merrill's in Boston, and Dr. Stanley Shaldon's in the UK, had begun dialyzing patients with chronic renal disease on a regular basis. But, many medical centers elsewhere had little interest in establishing dialysis programs for chronic kidney failure.

MY FELLOWSHIP YEARS in Dallas, under Donald W. Seldin, M.D. were some of the most valuable ones of my medical training. Dr. Seldin was, and at the time of this writing is, the quintessential teacher, researcher, and clinician. His clarity of thought, his vast knowledge of myriad subjects, and his logical summations of the salient aspects of any discussion were always exemplary. He was intimately involved with the research done by his fellows in training and always available to them for support and advice.

I also had the opportunity to work with Fredrik Kiil, M.D. (developer of the rebuildable parallel flow plate dialyzer) from Oslo, Norway, while he was in Dallas as visiting professor in the Department of Medicine. He too was involved in my basic research projects, as were Floyd Rector, Jr. M.D. and Norman

Carter, M.D., the other members of the Renal section. All were very generous of their time and knowledge. I welcomed the opportunity to study and learn in that environment.

During those years, I took every opportunity to gain as much practical clinical experience as I could. Since I had experience in cannulating blood vessels in my animal research, I was called on to insert arterial and venous catheters in patients who were undergoing hospital hemodialysis for acute kidney failure, from conditions such as poisonings, overdoses, and incompatible blood transfusions. Since I was available for this surgical procedure, the dialysis team didn't have to wait for the surgery resident to arrive before starting a dialysis.

I followed patients with chronic kidney failure in the Parkland Hospital out patient clinic and on hospital rounds. Many of these patients with chronic renal failure lived, for varying periods in reasonably stable states, with intermittent peritoneal dialysis. As their renal function inevitably worsened, intermittent dialysis no longer worked for them. When I left Dallas, in the summer of 1963, there were no established long-term dialysis programs for chronic progressive renal failure.

CHAPTER 5

PERITONEAL DIALYSIS

"In one case in the local women's clinic, where as a result of Uterine cancer, occlusion of the ureter(s) occurred (resulting in) acute uremia – so similar to our animal experiments.

I have infused 1½ liters of saline intraperitoneally. I had the impression that by making the infusion, the patient, already in Extremis has experienced a delay in the fatal outcome." **Georg Ganter: First use of peritoneal dialysis in a clinical situation. IWWM Vol 70: 1478-80. 1923,** *referenced from* **LIFE AND WORKS OF INTERNIST GEORG GANTER (1885-1940),** *with particular interest in (his) role in the history of peritoneal dialysis. Inaugural dissertation to the attainment of academic degree Dr. of Medicine. Diana Hess, presented 2010. Translated from the German.*

I wanted to offer Mrs. Kimble the option of peritoneal dialysis. I had no intention of starting a chronic dialysis program when I made this decision. I was particularly constrained in this matter, since, at that time, the Medical College of Georgia had neither chronic dialysis nor kidney transplant programs. In addition, none of the other hospitals in Augusta had any interest or capabilities of running a chronic dialysis program.

I considered dialysis a temporary measure to relieve a patient's uremic symptoms. It was feasible, that in a controlled environment, with fluid restriction, proper nutrition, and blood pressure control, Mrs. Kimble's renal function might improve enough that she could avoid further dialyses, at least temporarily. I thought back to patients in Dallas, who had often gone weeks between dialyses, and to the recent reports in the medical literature of patients with chronic renal failure surviving a month or longer between peritoneal dialyses. I was hoping that Mrs. Kimble might follow a similar course.

Mrs. Kimble had no medical insurance and little financial resources. She and her husband, partially disabled from a tractor accident in 1961, lived on their small farm in nearby Floyd County. Neither of them had finished high school, Mrs. Kimble finishing only the sixth grade. She told me they sharecropped their farm with a neighbor. They barely eked out a living.

The next day, Mrs. Kimble, four of her children, and her husband gathered in her hospital room. I explained to them the treatment option I wanted her to consider. "Mrs. Kimble," I began. "Your kidneys are badly damaged. They're unable to eliminate the toxic products that keep building up in your body and causing you to feel so miserable. But, there is a treatment called peritoneal dialysis, which can eliminate these poisons and bring you some relief." I explained exactly what the peritoneal dialysis procedure entailed. "After deadening an area in your abdominal wall with Novocaine, I will make a very small incision, about ¼ inch wide. Then, I will insert a small catheter through the incision into your belly. The catheter is hooked up to tubing connected to bottles of dialysis fluid. The fluid will then flow by gravity into your belly over a fifteen to twenty minute period. The fluid is left in for another sixty minutes or so, and then drained out. This procedure will be repeated until thirty-six exchanges have been made."

Mrs. Kimble had been listening very intently. She didn't seem unduly upset by my description of the procedure. Only asking, somewhat hesitantly, "Will it hurt very much, Doc?" Some of the children were shaking their heads, as if to imply they didn't want Mama to suffer through a process such as this.

"Mrs. Kimble, there will be a sensation of pressure as the fluid goes in, but if all goes as I expect, there should be little pain."

I gave the family and Mrs. Kimble a few minutes to talk amongst themselves before speaking again. "The sooner we begin, the better you will feel. Do you, or anyone, have any questions?"

"You sure this is going to help Mama?" Luke, the oldest of the children asked.

"Yes, I'm certain it will help." I turned to face Mrs. Kimble. "The question is for how long. The answer to that depends on how badly the kidneys are damaged. It also depends on how successful we are in controlling your blood pressure and certain other factors. You will need to be on a special diet with your fluids managed in such a manner that you become neither overloaded with fluid nor dehydrated. You will need to be very careful." I paused to let this sink in.

The children hovered around their mother's bed. All were talking at once—then a hush as Mrs. Kimble spoke. "Let's git on with it, Doc. Cain't be any worse than what I've been going through. Like I said before, I ain't been able to sleep for weeks. And I've got this awful taste in my mouth that I cain't get rid of, no matter how much I gargle with Listerine. Besides that, I've got this itch that jist won't stop. It's drivin' me crazy. Let's do that dialysis thing."

PERITONEAL DIALYSIS was used infrequently as a treatment option in Augusta at that time. It was not used to treat patients with chronic progressive kidney failure. I wanted to be sure that we had the proper dialysis solutions, tubing, catheter and other necessities for the dialysis, as well as the personnel to help run the exchanges. The hospital was able to locate a supplier who furnished the necessary equipment and supplies.

By the next morning, a private room was available for Mrs. Kimble. Special duty nurses were assigned to her for the duration of the treatment. The nursing staff was very cooperative in seeing that everything went smoothly.

We started early. The insertion of the catheter through the abdominal wall, via a trocar (a device ordinarily used for removing fluid from the peritoneal cavity) was surprisingly easy. I maneuvered it to a position as deep in the pelvic gutter as I could. I placed a sterile dressing around the catheter and taped it to her skin to keep it secure. The fluid exchanges went smoothly and Mrs. Kimble was even able to sleep for several hours during the procedure. She tolerated the fluid exchanges as though she'd experienced them a hundred times. She never complained. "I feel a lot better," she said, after the tenth exchange. We both were pleased.

I had spent the first two hours of the dialysis with Sally McKinnon, the RN assigned to Mrs. Kimble. Sally was twenty-one, smart, and efficient, a recent graduate of the University's Barrett School of Nursing. She and another RN, Jean Phillips, were assigned to manage the remainder of the dialysis procedure. Both nurses had helped me recently, when I used peritoneal dialysis for two patients with acute kidney failure. Those patients, fortunately, recovered their kidney function completely.

We finished Mrs. Kimble's dialysis the following day, around five in the afternoon. I had cut back my afternoon office schedule, so I could return to the hospital in time to check on the dialysis. After the thirty-sixth exchange, there was a decided improvement in her condition. Large amounts of excess fluid had been removed. Her breathing was now easy. She could lie flat in her bed. Even with the catheter still in place, Mrs. Kimble was smiling. "Where's the food, Doc?" she quipped. "I ain't been hungry like this in months." I slipped the catheter out slowly and closed the puncture wound with one silk stitch.

The next day, I called Dr. Mixon to give him a report on his patient. I was in the habit of sending patients back to their referring physician. Dr. Mixon, however, asked if I would continue to follow Mrs. Kimble on a regular basis. He said, since he had no experience with peritoneal dialysis, he would prefer that I follow her. I would then be in a better position to decide when she would need another dialysis.

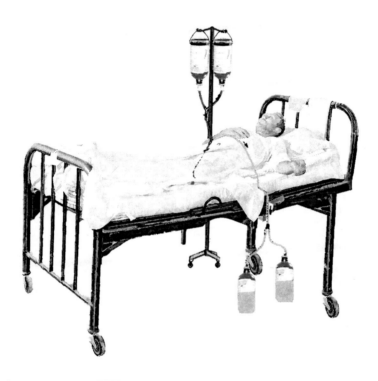

Peritoneal Dialysis Process

CHAPTER 6

THE DIET

For extreme diseases, extreme methods of cure, as to restriction, are most suitable. **APHORISMS of Hippocrates circa 400 B.C.E.** *Translated from the Greek by Francis Adams.*

Mrs. Kimble continued to feel "much better" throughout the day following her dialysis. I wanted to be sure that all her symptoms had abated and that her blood work and blood pressure were within a safe range. Additionally, I wanted to collect urines for creatinine clearances, (to measure more accurately her kidney function) and for the dietitian to instruct her, as to the type of foods she was to eat.

Low protein diets were introduced in the 1960s as a means of relieving uremic symptoms in those patients with chronic progressive renal failure. Also, it was hoped that these diets would slow down the rate of progression of chronic kidney failure. The Giordano/Giovannetti (G/G) diet from Italy, was the prototype.

The experiences of Doctors Sergio Giovannetti and Carmelo Giordano were quite impressive. The diet consisted of reducing the protein content to around 20 grams, limiting the sodium and potassium — when necessary — and insuring adequate calories and all the essential amino acids — the building blocks of proteins. In this manner, they were able to maintain a large number of severely impaired renal function patients free of uremic symptoms for extended periods of time — up to eighteen months in some cases.

I had asked Betty Simpson, RD, head dietitian at University Hospital, to study the G/G diet, and see if she might modify it in such a way that Mrs. Kimble felt comfortable following it, without changing the critical components of very low protein and, in her case, low salt and limited potassium.

Miss Simpson was very creative in modifying the diet specifically for Mrs. Kimble. Instead of emphasizing, as did the original diet, spaghetti made from wheat starch and bread made from maize starch, she allowed Mrs. Kimble more leeway.

She told her, "As long as you eat your 2 eggs each day and try to keep your protein level below 24 grams per day, you could even have a hot dog bun or a bagel from time to time. Think, especially, about getting the right amount of calories, which I've underlined on your diet plans. Eat the vegetables, fruits, and nuts that I've listed for you, and be very careful of those fruits and vegetables with high potassium."

As she did with the dialysis, Mrs. Kimble quickly adapted to the modified Giordano/Giovannetti diet. "Doc," she said, "I'm not used to this foreign food. I usually eat pancakes with Alaga syrup and bacon for breakfast, and now that diet lady tells me all I kin have is a grapefruit an' a piece of crumbly bread, with a dab of jelly! Don't know how I'll make it with no salt on my eggs though. S'pose I can git a'likin it, if I have to. If it's what I got to do to git well."

"Well, Mrs. Kimble," I said, "the name of the diet is foreign, but the foods Miss Simpson has selected for you are mostly American. You can have some bacon — thin crispy strips of the rinds would be best — and eggs, two a day. That's where you'll be getting most of your daily protein needs. One of the most important things is to be sure you eat all of the food on the diet each day. If not, your symptoms might come back."

"Doc, I'm gonna do the best I can. Sho' don't want to git sick agin, like I was." She smiled a bit.

After collecting urines for the clearances, and reviewing her blood tests, which were now in the safe range, I sat down by her bed and went over her treatment plan again. She was to keep a record of her weight each morning and measure and record her 24-hour urine volume daily. She was to adhere to the diet as closely as she could. I gave her prescriptions for multivitamins, Shohl's Solution (an alkalizing mixture similar to bicarbonate of soda, but with fewer side effects), and kept her on one blood pressure medication. I gave her an appointment to be seen in my office in one week. Since dialysis, her congestive state had improved markedly, but her BP was still not within the range I wanted.

After the dialysis, Mrs. Kimble's weight had dropped by some twelve pounds, all of which was excess fluid she needed to lose. I told her I wanted her weight to remain the same over the next week, even though I did not consider this to be her "dry weight," or a weight at which her congestive state — fluid overload — was corrected. I wanted to arrive at this goal slowly. She was to call me if any of her uremic symptoms recurred.

At her one-week post hospitalization office visit, Mrs. Kimble looked like a different person. Her nausea was gone. The skin lesions were healing. "My appetite is 'most back to normal," she volunteered. Her BP was still up a little, but well within an acceptable range. I made one adjustment in the dose of her blood pressure medication. I reassured her she was doing fine, and told her to continue her same regimen.

Over the next several months, Mrs. Kimble continued to improve. Her BP was brought under control and her kidneys showed some evidence of recovering a bit. Her clearances rose slightly, and on tight dietary protein restriction, all symptoms of uremia disappeared. She continued to lose more of her excess fluid, and her weight stabilized.

At her three months post dialysis visit, she weighed 110 pounds. I considered this her dry weight. Her appetite was good in spite of the dietary restrictions and lack of taste in many of her foods. At that time, her BP was fairly stable — 130/86. I had been able to more accurately follow her renal function by the 24-hour urines she brought with her at the time of her appointments. In the third month following her hospitalization, her clearances had improved modestly from the previous 4 ml/min to 7-8 ml/min, but still were drastically reduced. Her Hgb was about the same — 7.5 gm%. Mrs. Kimble was the patient most physicians dreamed of, compliant, considerate, and pleasant to be around, and she was responding to her treatment!

Her disabled husband, Herbert, had not been able to continue farming, and both he and Mrs. Kimble depended on what little financial assistance they received from her daughter, Evelyn. The Kimbles had fallen through the cracks of the state bureaucracy responsible for indigent people. They were told that, since they owned their house and their three-acre farm, they didn't qualify for public assistance. Life was difficult for the Kimbles. Money was scarce, and finding the necessary resources to buy some of the foods for her special diet was extremely worrisome and frustrating at times. But, Mrs. Kimble had managed to "feel good" most of the time. On her last office visit, she told me, "I'm stayin' on that diet, Doc. It's tough, but so far, I think I've done a pretty good job of it. I've made a little money selling eggs. You know, I got twelve layin' hens. Every little bit helps. My daughter, Evelyn, helps me with my grocery shopping and around the house, when she can take the time away from tendin' to her own chill'un and husband."

The Kimbles, of course, still had no hospitalization insurance. I was concerned as to how University Hospital would react when Mrs. Kimble needed another dialysis, which I felt certain she would need eventually. I was hoping they would allow me to admit her electively, about every three weeks — the interval I anticipated might be necessary between dialyses. I felt that her age precluded her from being a realistic candidate for kidney transplantation. I never expected her to be free of uremic symptoms and doing this well with the diet alone — for this long.

IT HAD BEEN a little more than six months since Mrs. Kimble's hospitalization, and she continued to keep her regular office appointments with me. Her renal clearances had not improved during this period, but they had held steady, in the range of 7-8 ml/min. Her Hgb remained around 8 gm%, but her endurance was "better than it used to be." She was going about her usual household chores, preparing meals for her husband, sweeping and mopping floors, doing the laundry, and occasionally "jist sitting around and doing nothin." Still, she hadn't required another dialysis.

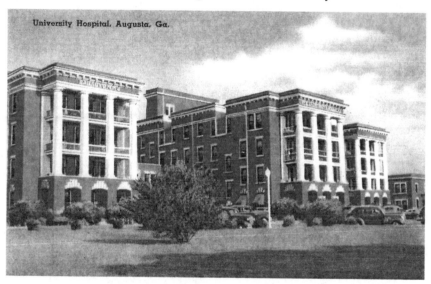

University Hospital, Augusta, Ga.

Postcard of the old University Hospital

CHAPTER 7

JIMMY WELLS

"It is, indeed, an humiliating confession, that, although much attention has been directed to this disease for nearly ten years, and during that time there has probably been no period in which at least twenty cases might not have been pointed out in each of the large hospitals of the metropolis (London)... yet little or nothing has been done toward devising a method of permanent relief, when the disease has been confirmed; and no fixed plan has been laid down, as affording a tolerable certainty of cure ..." **Bright, Richard, Guy's Hospital Reports, 1827, vol 1, p. 93 from Original Papers of Richard Bright on Renal Disease Ed. A. Arnold Osman, D.S.C., F.R.C.P. Oxford University Press, 1937**

Along with Mrs. Kimble, I had been following a number of other patients with chronic renal disease. All were on the modified Giovannetti/Giordano diet and, with the exception of a young man named Jimmy Wells, none had reached the end stage of kidney failure. All were doing well, with good blood pressure and weight control.

Jimmy was a twenty one year old, ex college student, who carried the diagnosis of chronic glomerular nephritis. Dr. Raymond Billingsley asked me to see Jimmy in consultation. Dr. Billingsley, a busy GP in Mill Valley, SC, had been following Jimmy for the last ten years, since he first discovered albumin (frequently a harbinger of progressive renal failure) in his urine.

Dr. Billingsley had admitted Jimmy because he was becoming uremic. His BUN had been rising gradually over the last several years and was now hovering around 150 mg%. He had become anemic, with Hgb levels in the 8 gm% range. His appetite was poor and he had bouts of nausea on a daily basis. His BP was still elevated, even though he was on several antihypertensive drugs.

Jimmy was a little over six feet tall, with short cropped, scraggly, blond hair. His face was sallow and puffy. He was short of breath as he walked from his chair to a bed for me to examine him.

Jimmy was suffering from the effects of chronic renal failure. In his case, as in that of Mrs. Kimble, I wanted to relieve his uremic symptoms before deciding on a long-term treatment plan. Initially, I didn't go into detail with him about his condition, except to explain that because of his failing kidneys, there was an accumulation of toxic products in his body. I also informed him that we needed to perform a procedure, peritoneal dialysis, to rid him of these products as soon as possible. During that hospital admission, Jimmy underwent a 36-hour peritoneal dialysis. He tolerated the procedure, without complaining and without complications.

The following day, after the dialysis, he was feeling "much better." I sat on the edge of his bed and asked him to tell me a bit more about himself. I asked how he'd been feeling, and what he'd been doing in the several months prior to this admission. His sister, Nettie, an LPN at University, sat in a recliner next to his bed. Before he had a chance to speak, she offered, "Jimmy's always had a good appetite, so when he would just leave, sometimes, over half of the meal I fixed, I knew something was wrong. Sometimes he would leave the table, because the smell of food made him nauseous."

Jimmy said, "Doc, I guess you know, I just finished my junior year at USC, Aiken, this spring and—"

Nettie interrupted, "and, Doc, for three years Jimmy was a first string pitcher for his team, until his kidneys quit working right."

"I tried to finish out this season, Doc," Jimmy continued, "but I started gettin' tired, after I'd pitched about three or four innings. And whenever I'd get tired, I'd most always get nauseated. Then, we were playin' Newcombe Valley—it was our third game of the season—and I had to ask coach Davis to take me out. I walked over to the bench and threw up. That was the last time I was able to play."

"I got really depressed after that—thinkin' that I might not ever be able to play baseball again. I wasn't even thinkin' about my kidneys gettin' worse at that time. Ya' see, I'd known I had bad kidneys ever since I was a kid, but they never gave me any trouble until this year. When Dr. Billingsley told me they were gettin' worse and he wanted me to see you, I never really gave much thought to them really quitin' on me. I thought there must be somethin' that could be done to get them workin' right again. I never really thought they were goin' to eventually give out."

Jimmy, and his sister, two years older, lived with their mother in Mill Valley, South Carolina. Mrs. Wells was a widow and had a steady job at the Baker Brothers Mill, the one job producing business in that part of Johnson County. The mill did provide a very limited amount of hospital insurance for Mrs. Wells, but it was not a family policy and didn't cover Jimmy.

Jimmy was nearing, or had already had arrived at, end stage kidney disease. I arranged to have the dietitian talk with him, his mother, and his sister before he was discharged. Because of his lack of insurance coverage and scanty financial resources, Jimmy's hospitalization was kept as brief as possible, without compromising his safety. I didn't undertake to measure his creatinine clearances because of these circumstances. I planned to collect the 24-hour urines and blood work needed for such calculations, as an outpatient.

On the day of his discharge, I discussed with Jimmy, his mother, and Nettie what I felt we had to offer him. "Jimmy, I know you're used to living with the knowledge that your kidneys were damaged. Dr. Billingsley told me he explained to you that they had reached a point where the damage was so severe; he didn't know what else he could do to improve their function. And he's right, if we're talking about doing something to correct the damage that's already been done. But, there is something that can be done, which may help you live a better life with your damaged kidneys. Until we can make arrangements for you to have a kidney transplant. That something is called peritoneal dialysis."

"You mean that treatment I just got through with, Doc?"

"Yes, it would mean coming back into the hospital periodically and flushing out the poisons with another dialysis. In addition, there's a new diet that two Italian researchers, Drs. Giovannetti and Giordano, have had real success with in treating patients with your type of kidney disease. So, I'm going to suggest we begin both programs — peritoneal dialysis and that special diet. The diet you will receive is a modification of the Italian one — for American tastes.

"Both peritoneal dialysis and this new, very low protein diet have the potential for relieving most of the symptoms you've been having. Eventually, you'll become stabilized, be able to eat without feeling nauseated, and have more energy. Meanwhile, we'll search diligently for a facility that will accept you for a kidney transplant. To my way of thinking, a kidney transplant offers you the best opportunity to live a more normal life. The diet and peritoneal dialyses are temporary measures to relieve your symptoms — and to keep you going."

'But doctor," Mrs. Wells interjected, "we just don't have the money for all this. How can we afford it?"

"I realize, Mrs. Wells, that University Hospital may have a problem admitting Jimmy without hospital insurance. But I'm hoping they will, if I can find a way to supply the dialysis solutions and equipment."

I had a plan—although not completely worked out in my mind—to discuss Jimmy's case with a friend of mine, Bill Sessions, at Baxter/Travenol, a medical supply company. I hoped that after hearing about Jimmy's condition, his lack of hospital insurance, and his desperate financial status, Bill would be willing to furnish the equipment and supplies for dialysis treatments at no charge.

In my short time in private practice, I had found representatives of pharmaceutical and medical supply companies, to be very responsive to the needs of indigent patients. They were often willing to supply them with free drugs, medical supplies, and even, on occasion, medical equipment.

I told Jimmy that once he started dialysis, I would expect him to be admitted to the hospital, every three weeks, for a day and a half. I was hoping Jimmy could stay on his diet and we could control his blood pressure. If so, he might get by with such a dialysis schedule—or maybe with an even longer interval between dialyses.

When I finished talking with the Wells' family, I felt that each of them understood what following this program would mean for Jimmy. In addition to returning to the hospital every three weeks, he would be expected to stay on a very restricted diet: low sodium, low protein and low potassium. I felt reasonably confident that I would be able to acquire the necessary dialysis supplies and equipment for him. I was less confident as to how the University Hospital would react, when I explained the care Jimmy would need, and about his ability to accept this new lifestyle.

CHAPTER 8

ADMINISTRATION

University Hospital was built in 1915, replacing Augusta's City and Lamar hospitals. The new hospital featured two symmetrical wings. The Barrett wing served "White" patients and the Lamar wing the city's "Colored" patients. All areas were desegregated starting in 1965, following passage of the Civil Rights Act of 1964.

Early the next week, I met with Adam Higgans, the Assistant Administrator of University Hospital, in his office. Adam was in his mid thirties. He was tall, thin, with a receding hairline, and soft spoken. I had gotten along well with him. He was always very reasonable, understanding, and most of all, a patient advocate.

"I appreciate your taking the time to see me," I began. "Jimmy Wells, the patient I want to talk to you about, lives in South Carolina—Johnson County. He has chronic kidney failure and was hospitalized here last week. At that time, we performed peritoneal dialysis, and—"

"Yes, Doctor, I know about Jimmy, his condition, and his family. I've read your hospital consultation report and the hospital discharge summary. I've talked with the Wells family, and I've been wanting to talk with you about this case."

"Then I can get straight to the point," I said. "To put it bluntly, if he is unable to receive regular dialyses, his prognosis is dismal. The peritoneal dialysis he underwent during his initial hospitalization went very smoothly. Right now, he is free of symptoms from his kidney failure, but because his kidneys are chronically damaged, inevitably, his symptoms will return. If he's to survive, he will need some sort of dialytic support."

"This too, I understand," Mr. Higgans nodded.

I continued, "I was hoping to persuade the administration to allow Jimmy to come in for peritoneal dialysis on a regular basis — say, every three weeks — at least initially."

"The problem is," Mr. Higgans replied, "Jimmy has no hospitalization insurance. He's a South Carolina resident, and it's our understanding that the family is on welfare. I'm afraid it will be very difficult for us to agree on a regular admitting schedule for Mr. Wells."

"Mr. Higgans, you know, being proactive in managing patients with chronic kidney failure is a new approach to treating this condition. Ten years ago — no, even six or five years ago — a patient with Jimmy's condition would have had no hope of staying alive. Now, a few centers are beginning to dialyze such patients, and they are surviving longer. Transplantation programs are being developed along with these dialysis programs. I'm sure you're aware of these new happenings in medicine."

"Yes, I have been reading about these developments in your field, Doctor. Of course, you know that we, as a community hospital, are in no position to think about starting such programs here."

"I understand your position completely. But the arrangement I would like you to consider is this: Set aside a room for dialysis. Maybe on Barrett 2, but any space would be acceptable with me. I will arrange for private duty nurses, with peritoneal dialysis experience, to monitor the procedure, after I start it. Also, I will arrange for the supplies and equipment necessary for the dialysis, at no cost to the hospital. Total time for one dialysis will ordinarily be less than forty hours. In essence, hospital expenses would be limited to the use of one room for two days, and hopefully, only every three weeks until ... well, I'm not sure when. Jimmy is certainly a candidate for a kidney transplant. I've already begun making enquiries around the country for a program that will accept him."

I knew Mr. Higgans was aware of Jimmy's deteriorating condition. Also, I was hoping he was doing some soul searching about a community's obligation to its fellow citizens. Then too, he had a responsibility to the institution he represented. He was listening intently to my proposition.

I kept talking. "The Medical College of Georgia is planning to do kidney transplants in the not too distant future. I know this because of conversations I've had with several of my colleagues at MCG. So, if Jimmy and other patients with chronic kidney failure can be dialyzed and stay healthy, they should be candidates for a kidney transplant soon."

"Doctor, thanks for the in-service," he chuckled. "I like your proposal. Personally, I want to help Jimmy Wells. I'll certainly make a strong case for the arrangement you've suggested, when I bring this up with my boss, Mr. Harris."

I felt Mr. Harris, likely, would go along with my proposal. He depended a great deal on Higgans' recommendations concerning the day-to-day management of hospital affairs, as well as his assessment of when to add new services or delete old ones. I was confident that Baxter/Travenol would do their part.

CHAPTER 9

CHALLENGES

"The most important limiting factors for long term peritoneal dialysis are: 1) pain during dialysis and 2) infections (peritonitis) followed by adhesions." **Vol X Trans. American Society Artif. Organs 1964; S.T.Boen et al.**

Soon after I started practice in Augusta, I began depositing the stipend I received as Medical Director of the University Hospital Outpatient Clinic in a separate *Kidney Account*. Also, I deposited a percentage of the income from my general medical practice in that account. I used withdrawals exclusively for patients with chronic kidney disease, and to help pay for these patients' medications, blood work, and later expenses for dialysis.

As it turned out, University Hospital continued to provide some of the nursing support for Jimmy Wells' dialysis treatments. My office nurse, Jeannie Carter, worked with the hospital based dialysis nursing team. Jeannie was a LPN trained under the University Hospital program. She was skilled in all the nursing aspects of peritoneal dialysis — and later hemodialysis — and was extremely competent in instilling confidence and hope in her patients.

I was admitting Jimmy for his fifth dialytic treatment. Baxter/Travenol, as part of their service to indigent patients, arranged to provide the equipment and supplies for his dialyses. University in turn, agreed to admit him, when he needed dialysis treatments.

Administration set aside a room in the hospital, on Barrett 2, for dialysis, a room that would not require sacrificing space for general medical or surgical patients. It had been used as a treatment area for administering intravenous drugs, performing specialized diagnostic procedures, physical examinations, and such. A curtain partitioned the room, and even on those days when dialysis was performed, it could still be used for those special procedures.

Prior to this admission, Jimmy's dialyses had lasted thirty-six hours, with a three-week interval between them. I was hoping this schedule would allow him enough respite from his uremia to achieve a decent quality of life. My experience with Mrs. Kimble gave me a reason to be hopeful.

In the short term, the dialyses were very effective in relieving Jimmy's symptoms, but three weeks between them proved too long. He had much difficulty following the protein and salt restricted diet. He had trouble, especially, limiting his fluids. His uremic symptoms began reappearing, usually, by the end of the second week post dialysis. On each hospital admission, he was "feeling miserable."

This admission was no exception. He was nauseous, bloated, itched severely, and had markedly elevated blood pressures. His creatinine clearances were averaging 5 ml/min. — dangerously low. I lengthened his dialysis time from thirty-six to forty-eight hours, hoping this would result in some abatement of his uremic symptoms between dialyses. I was reluctant to suggest a more frequent schedule, for obvious reasons: the commitments I had made to University Hospital, and the one to Jimmy about a dialysis treatment every three weeks. I did not want to test University's resolve of continuing to care for him, or his resolve to continue coming for dialysis treatments, by insisting on more frequent dialyses. I felt this was the best we could do for him, considering the circumstances. I worried that lengthening the hospitalization time for him might be a problem for the hospital administration.

When I made the decision to dialyze Jimmy, I viewed peritoneal dialysis as a diagnostic/therapeutic maneuver to relieve his uremic state, and to afford us an opportunity to evaluate his underlying kidney reserve. He might even do as well as Mrs. Kimble. Maybe he would stabilize with the diet and infrequent dialyses. At worst, this regimen would be a stopgap measure, until a kidney transplant program accepted him.

Academic centers had either started or were considering starting chronic dialysis programs. Emory, in Atlanta, had begun dialyzing a small number of patients with chronic renal failure on a regular basis and was starting a renal transplant program. Moreover, a few other centers around the country were beginning kidney transplant programs. The Medical College of Georgia was still several years away from establishing such programs. The chances of one of these new, or older, programs accepting Jimmy were slim. Few had the space or resources to take on additional patients from outside their immediate referral base.

Unfortunately, although not surprisingly, lengthening Jimmy's time on dialysis proved ineffective in mitigating his uremic symptoms. During his time at home, between dialyses, he became depressed, and at times, almost despondent. At a visit to my office, he told me, "Doc, I can't keep going on this way. I feel terrible most of the time. For a few days, after I finish a dialysis, I feel like I might can make it 'till the time for my next dialysis, but then, in about a week, it hits me again — all the bad feelings. I got now, where I just dread coming in for my dialysis."

Jimmy was not staying on his diet. He was becoming withdrawn from his friends and from his family. He tolerated his dialyses less and less. Now, he dreaded "being stuck." At each dialysis, I had to make a small incision in his abdominal wall, in order to insert the trochar — and later a specially designed stylet catheter. The procedure of catheter insertion, which initially had caused minimal discomfort, now was creating anxiety, pain, and fear of pain as the catheter was maneuvered into place in his peritoneal cavity. These feelings were exacerbated by his uremic state. Jimmy always sensed pressure as the peritoneum was punctured, but until the last several dialyses, he didn't complain of any significant pain. Now, he became very anxious as the abdominal area was prepped for the catheter insertion. He would become distraught and agitated. He had convinced himself that he couldn't tolerate continuing with the dialyses. Something had to change.

CHAPTER 10

BUTTONS

"A subcutaneous peritoneal access button has been used clinically for two years. No serious complications have been encountered." A **Clinically Successful Subcutaneous Peritoneal Access Button for Repeated Peritoneal Dialysis. Vol. X; 1964 Trans. Amer. Soc. Artif. Organs. W. G. Mallette, et al**

While doing my research in Dallas, conducting animal (dog) studies, I used Teflon "buttons" shaped in the form of a hollow spool. I needed to collect urine separately from each kidney. This was accomplished by splitting the animal's bladder in half. The button was sutured in place in each hemi-bladder. Urine, then, was easily obtained, separately from each kidney.

The idea of using buttons, such as these, for patients needing dialysis, was first suggested to me by Norman Carter, M.D. He and his research group were studying salt wasting in patients with chronic renal disease at that time. Some of these patients had been receiving dialysis by the intermittent puncture technique; and he was looking for a more efficient method of dialyzing. Later, for a short period, Norman's group did use implanted buttons of different designs, in a number of patients with chronic renal failure. Other groups used plastic or Teflon conduits and buttons implanted between the abdominal cavity and the skin.

In Augusta, I modified the design of the buttons I had used in Dallas, and the Department of Surgery at MCG made a prototype for me. I planned to use this button on Jimmy Wells, in the hope of relieving some of his discomfort and anxiety.

The method of using a button for dialysis, was to surgically implant it, below the umbilicus, through the skin, subcutaneous tissue, and musculature with the lower portion of the device being maneuvered through a small opening in the peritoneum. The upper portion was positioned immediately beneath the skin.

Theoretically, after the incision for placing the button had healed, the skin over the button should slip easily over the top of the button. Then a small incision would be made in the skin, as usual, and the catheter introduced through the opening in the middle of the button, and into the peritoneal cavity. At each subsequent dialysis, a new small stab wound would be made in the skin, at a slightly different site, for the insertion of the catheter.

By having this button in place in the lower abdominal wall, the peritoneal cavity could be entered repeatedly, and the dialysis solutions introduced in a non-traumatic manner. I explained to Jimmy that I would like to use this button for his dialyses. I told him that, by eliminating the puncture of the peritoneal membrane, he should be able to tolerate the dialytic procedure with less pain and discomfort.

Jimmy wasn't pleased about undergoing the surgery required for implanting the button. He told me, "I'm willing to give this button a try if you're sure it will make me feel any better."

I explained, "The surgery will be minimal and can actually be done without putting you to sleep. It should take no more than thirty to forty minutes. I do believe using the button will reduce some of the discomfort you're having now."

I arranged for Jimmy's admittance directly from my office. I wanted to begin the dialysis in the usual manner, but I told him that I would see to it that he was given enough medication to ease his anxiety and pain. Following the dialysis, he was to have the necessary surgery for the implanting of the button.

Dr. Harry Sherman, a general and vascular surgeon, and a friend and colleague, implanted the button, following Jimmy's dialysis. There were no complications and Jimmy was discharged the next day.

Since, he was becoming uremic between dialyses, and since the increased time on dialysis had not changed his clinical course in a positive way, I felt obligated to have him return for dialysis more frequently. I persuaded him to come for dialysis every two, instead of three weeks. I emphasized that the button would make the treatments much more bearable, and that the more frequent dialyses should relieve many of his uremic symptoms. I hoped University Hospital would not object to our changing his treatment plan. Fortunately, they didn't.

At this early stage in the evolution of dialysis for chronic renal failure, there were no clearly established criteria for frequency of dialysis. But, those who were trying to manage these patients were quickly finding out how long individual patients could forego dialyzing. At that time, it was not so much finding the optimum interval between dialyses. It was more like, how long we can put off dialyzing without endangering, or composing the quality of our patients' lives.

From the perspective of twenty-first century medical practices, such an approach to managing a sick patient seems inadequate, to say the least. In the 1960s, circumstances dictated different approaches to caring for patients with chronic kidney disease. Funding for treatment was practically non-existent, except at some academic facilities. Many patients had no hospitalization insurance, and those who did, usually found that any sort of dialysis was not a covered treatment. Medicaid was just being implemented and unevenly administered. Medicare had not begun to cover dialysis treatments for chronic renal failure.

Indigent patients were seldom turned away from hospitals for ordinary sicknesses or injuries. However, city/county, religious, or other privately run hospitals were not willing to assume the financial risks associated with treating patients with chronic progressive kidney failure. These patients might need treatment for months, if not years, awaiting a kidney transplant.

Most of my patients with kidney problems came to me through referrals. Many times, at least early on, referred patients with chronic renal failure were relatively young. Many of them had diagnosed kidney disease, and their referring doctor had been following them for years.

Historically, treatment for patients with chronic progressive kidney failure had been palliative, which, in reality, meant making them as comfortable as possible until they died. Managing them was much like current hospice programs.

However, in the decade of the 1960s, doctors and patients were learning quickly of these more progressive treatments for kidney failure. The demands and referrals for these services were increasing.

When Jimmy returned for his next dialysis, the incision site over the button had not healed completely. I was unable to use the button. I elected to administer enough medication to assuage his anxiety, and to start the dialysis in the usual manner, by the intermittent puncture technique.

Other than waking briefly for food and water, he slept through the entire procedure. The incision over the button showed no evidence of infection, and it was healing nicely. Hopefully, I could use the button for his next treatment.

At home, Jimmy still was not doing well, and remained depressed. Nettie kept me informed. Early one morning when I was making rounds at the hospital, she stopped me. "Doc, I just can't get Jimmy to cut out his Pepsi drinks. I think he may be hooked on 'em. He's drinking maybe eight to ten a day. And he refuses to take his blood pressure medications regularly. He knows that's just making everythin' much worse. We've got those scales you told us to get, and I've been keepin' a record of his weight every day. And, of course, it's not anywhere close to the number you told us it should be. It's just got where, it looks like he doesn't seem to care anymore about what's good for himself."

I told Nettie that I would talk with Jimmy when he came in for his next dialysis, and encourage him to make a more concerted effort to stay on his diet and to limit his fluids.

All the while, I was searching for transplant programs. The Medical College of Virginia, in Richmond, was one of the few programs that offered some hope. They placed Jimmy on their waiting list, but implied that the chances were poor that he would be accepted soon. Nettie was the only possible donor. She was ready and willing to be tested. Some cadaveric transplants were being performed, following the first one in Boston in 1962. However, acceptance for a cadaver transplant was an even more remote possibility for Jimmy.

It was Friday and Jimmy had been admitted to the hospital for his regular treatment. We had been using his dialysis button for the last two months. He was tolerating the dialysis procedure a little better now, and said his pain was less. He was definitely less apprehensive. But, as we prepped his abdomen for the insertion of the catheter, he said to me, "I've come to hate this whole thing of peritoneal dialysis, Doc, and I don't know how much longer I can put up with it."

Jimmy had been having regular dialysis treatments now, for almost eight months, but remained under dialyzed. His symptoms, as well as his blood work, reflected this. The dialysis exchanges were going smoothly, once the catheter was in place, but the button was not the solution I hoped it to be. I began having trouble getting the skin to slip smoothly over it. Finding a new, not inflamed or scarred area of skin, in which to make the small incision, was becoming more and more difficult. During his last dialysis, I had to make the incision so far from the button that the catheter kept kinking. I had to insert another catheter before finally getting the dialysis fluid to flow properly.

Because of these complications with inserting the catheter via the button, and because Jimmy was becoming very despondent, I had real concerns that time was running out for him.

Dialyzing every two weeks did not relieve his uremic symptoms for long. I knew Jimmy wouldn't agree to more frequent dialyses. He had told me so in no uncertain terms. I knew, even if he had agreed to more time, I would have difficulty convincing University Hospital to cover more frequent or longer treatments.

Shortly after we started the dialysis, I sat on the foot of his bed. Leaning over, I rested my hand on his knee. "Jimmy", I said, "listen, I hear what you're saying. You know, I'm still trying to find additional transplant programs that will put you on their waiting list. The dialyses will keep you going until a spot on one of those programs opens up. I don't know how long that will be. But, if you can just try harder to stay on your diet, I can promise that your symptoms will lessen."

"Doc" he replied, "this life I got has got me down. I kinda lost my spirit. Right after I have my dialysis, I try to get out of the house and see some of my old friends. They encourage me to come see 'em." He hesitated, his voice was barely audible, tears welled up in his eyes. "Doc, you just don't know how tough it is, having to live like an invalid. I never feel good enough to do much of anythin'. I never know when I'm gonna be nauseated. I'm always afraid of throwin' up when I'm around people. I'm sick of it—sick of it, Doc. Do you understand?" He held his head in his hands and began sobbing, almost silently. Tears rolled down his cheeks. I did my best to comfort him. But Jimmy was exhausted physically and mentally. He deserved better.

CHAPTER 11

COMPLICATIONS

"... in some patients in chronic renal failure, potassium intoxication was a problem; the less severe uremics were able to excrete potassium in adequate amounts so as to prevent harmful retention." **Diet in Chronic Uremia. S. Giovannetti. Proc. 3rd Congress Nephrology, Washington, 1966, Vol. 3: p 235**

I had been seeing Rita Kimble regularly every month. She was staying on her diet with an almost religious determination. Her kidney function was basically unchanged. Her creatinine clearances had dropped slightly, and now varied between 4 and 5 ml/min — a precarious level, but one which allowed her to continue going about her life as she had before becoming severely uremic some ten months ago.

On this visit, as on each of her previous appointments, Mrs. Kimble brought me a dozen eggs, "compliments of my hens," she said. She left a basket of "just picked tomatoes" for my secretary and nurse. Although we never discussed her bill — which I had stopped sending and had already written off — bringing these gifts was her way, in some small measure, of helping to pay for her care. She had driven alone the thirty or so miles from her house to my office. She looked good and had no complaints. Her blood pressure was normal, and she had no swelling of the feet or elsewhere. Her blood work was decent. Her weight was exactly where I wanted it to be.

"Mrs. Kimble," I said, "as long as you're doing this well without dialysis, I see no need to change anything. Just continue everything you're doing."

She left in good humor, thanking our office staff for "being so nice."

Three weeks after Mrs. Kimble's last visit, I received a telephone call from her son Luke. It was early in the morning and I was leaving home to make hospital rounds. He told me they rushed his mother to Floyd County Hospital the previous night. She had become extremely weak, and had fallen getting out of the bathtub. He said, "She didn't break any bones, Doc, but she's pretty bruised up and sore."

I told Luke how sorry I was to hear that, and I would contact the doctors at Floyd County to check on her as soon as I got to my office. Before I left the house, my home phone rang again. It was my answering service giving me a number to call at Floyd County Hospital. The call was from Dr. Nelson Bennett, a friend of mine, working in the ER there last night.

"George," Nelson began, "your patient, Rita Kimble, was brought to our ER around ten last night. Apparently, she got extremely weak after taking a hot bath and fell getting out of the tub, injuring her elbows and right hip. She has contusions over her hip, arms, and thighs, but luckily, no fractures. Her initial serum potassium was elevated — 6.5, and her EKG showed peaked T waves. I was concerned that the high potassium might have been responsible for a cardiac arrhythmia, leading to the weakness and subsequent fall. I went ahead and gave her a Kayexalate enema. We've repeated her electrolytes and her potassium is back to normal." He continued, "Mrs. Kimble told us you had her on a very strict diet for her chronic kidney condition. In fact, she brought a copy of it with her. She said she didn't want to bother you last night, but would like us to call you today, and let you know she's in our hospital. And that you shouldn't worry, she was sticking to her diet."

I said, "Yeah, that sure sounds like Mrs. Kimble. She never wants to put anybody out."

"Today, her vital signs are stable," Nelson continued. "Her BUN, of course, is still elevated. We're gonna patch her up a bit, and if this meets with your approval, ask her to make an appointment with you for follow up."

"That's fine with me, Nelson. Tell her to call my office when she gets home. And thanks for taking care of her. Give me a call next time you're in town, and maybe we can get together, at least for lunch."

I too, was concerned that Mrs. Kimble's weakness and subsequent fall might have been triggered by a cardiac arrhythmia. High blood potassium levels can cause disturbances in cardiac function and subsequent blood pressure drops. I knew Mrs. Kimble was aware of this danger. Betty Simpson, the dietitian at University, had warned her to be especially careful when it came to eating vegetables or fruit with high potassium content.

Two days later, when I saw Mrs. Kimble in my office, she was still "very sore" and moved about cautiously. Other than that, she had no complaints, and was her usual cheery self.

"You been doin' alright, Doc?" she asked. "I was worried about them botherin' you th' night I went to Floyd County hospital. That's why I didn't want 'em to call you, at least until more civilized hours."

"Well, Mrs. Kimble, I appreciate your concern, but as I've said before, any time you get to feeling like something's not going right with you, I want, and expect, you to give me a call. I'm just glad that you didn't break any bones in your fall."

"Doc, Dr. Bennett, at Floyd, asked me a lot about the foods I've been eatin'. He seemed concerned, like maybe, I'd been eatin' too many tomatoes. I haf' to admit, that since our garden came in a couple of weeks ago, I probably haf' been eatin' more of them than I should of. I love fresh tomatoes."

"You just have to be more careful about the tomatoes, and potatoes, and squash. I believe you told me that those were some of your favorites. Right?"

"You're right, Doc. I know what I should eat, but every now and then I get to thinkin' how good a fresh tomato with mayonnaise on white bread would taste, and I'll admit, I likely ate a few more uh them than I should of."

"Well, you're human," I smiled. "Just be extra careful now."

I drew blood for a check on her electrolytes—which includes potassium levels. Later that day, I received the report, and all values were back to normal. I called Mrs. Kimble at home the next day, and told her the potassium was okay. I knew I didn't have to remind her to be careful with all those good, fresh vegetables around, but I did.

CHAPTER 12

ROBERT JACKSON

"Headache is the most common presenting symptom of hypertensive encephalopathy, followed by seizures, focal neurological deficits and loss of consciousness." **Nervenarzt, August 2010; 81(B) Headache and Hypertension. Myth and evidence. T. Liman, et al**

Malignant Hypertension refers to the syndrome of severely elevated blood pressure, retinal changes, including papilledema (swelling of the optic disc) and hemorrhages, renal dysfunction, and hypertensive encephalopathy. This is not a cancer or neoplastic disorder, but carries a very poor prognosis none the less. Life expectancy without treatment usually is rarely over one year.

In earlier days, with the antihypertensive drugs then available, treatment of this condition was never completely satisfactory. Surgical procedures, such as sympathectomy (removing all or portions of a patient's autonomic nervous system, responsible for the fight or flight responses) were used with some success, but often with severe side effects.

In the 1940s, and on into the '50s, '60s, and early '70s, Walter Kempner, at Duke, treated thousands of hypertensive patients with his rice diet. Dr. Kempner had remarkable success with his treatment protocol. Those patients, who could stay on his extremely rigid program of salt and protein restriction for long periods, frequently evidenced significant, and long lasting, improvement in renal function, reversal of their eye ground changes, reductions in blood pressure to normal levels, and resolution of cardiac dysfunction.

Before Kempner's approach to treating malignant hypertension, the changes in the eye grounds and kidneys, as well as the elevated blood pressure, were considered irreversible. As Dr. Kempner pointed out, in an address given to the American College of Physicians, on March 30, 1949, "The important result is not that the change in the course of the disease has been achieved by the rice diet, but that the course of the disease can be changed."

I was aware of Dr. Kempner's work, even before I entered medical school. My uncle, Frank S. Van Giesen, of Savannah, who was diagnosed with chronic nephritis and severe hypertension, was a regular patient of Kempner in the 1940s and early '50s.

I recall my grandmother speaking to my father, "Frank's gone to Duke again. He's off his diet. He says it's making him crazy. I know his blood pressure's sure to go up now."

My uncle lived for many years while on — and off — the rice diet, but eventually succumbed to his chronic Bright's disease at age fifty, in an era before dialysis and transplantation.

During the sixties, newer and more potent drugs were available, resulting in less emphasis on dietary measures for this devastating condition. Gradually, the rice diet lost its place in the armamentarium for treating malignant hypertension.

MY MEDICAL PRACTICE was growing. I was being asked to see patients for medical evaluation prior to surgery, and was acquiring new patients on self-referral, as well as on physician referral. But, I was spending much of my time with my kidney patients, especially my patients with chronic kidney dysfunction.

I first met Robert Jackson in April of 1967, while he was in University Hospital, under the care of Dr. Steve Springer, the Neurologist who had admitted him for seizures.

Dr. Springer's workup had revealed no evidence of a brain tumor or other primary neurological disorder. He had concluded that Robert's seizures were related to his malfunctioning kidneys. His diagnoses were encephalopathy with seizures, secondary to malignant hypertension, secondary to chronic renal failure. He asked me to see Robert in consultation.

Robert was twenty years old. Two years ago, he had graduated from Laney High School, a black only school in Augusta. Since his graduation, he had been working regularly, as a delivery driver for Hurst Brothers Bread Company. Fortunately for him, his first seizure occurred while he was home, getting ready for work.

Robert lived with his grandmother, who had raised him. He never knew his father. His mother died at childbirth after delivering a stillborn. His grandmother was devoted to him as he was to her. The only symptoms he had experienced prior to his seizures were occasional nausea, mild fatigue, some blurring of his vision on occasions, and headaches that worsened when he exerted himself. He admitted that the headaches were happening more frequently over the last several months.

His past medical history was relatively benign. He'd never been hospitalized, and only saw doctors on infrequent occasions: once, after a fall from his bicycle when he was four, and with a "bad strep throat." He'd never been told there was anything wrong with his kidneys.

On my examination, I found Robert's blood pressure to be above 220/126 on repeated checks. Clinically, and by X-ray, his heart was markedly enlarged, his neck veins were prominent, there was a puffiness about his face, and some mild swelling of the feet. His urine gave a strong reaction for protein, and large numbers of renal failure casts were seen in the urinary sediment. On X-ray, the kidneys were symmetrically reduced in size.

The most striking features of my exam were in his eyes. Ordinarily, when viewing normal eye grounds — ophthalmoscopy — one is able to see the central retinal disc with clear margins and good pulsations of the small veins of the retina. Robert's retinal picture was totally altered. The central disc was completely blurred — papilledema. There were no venous pulsations, and there were extensive hemorrhages and exudates throughout.

Robert's renal function was compromised. His BUN was 110 mg% and Creatinine 8 mg%, at the time of admission. His Hgb was 9. Dr. Springer had placed Robert on several antihypertensive medications prior to my consultation, but they had done little to reduce his blood pressure.

I was concerned with Robert's BP still being dangerously high. I ordered 2.5 mg. of intramuscular Reserpine, a drug I had used in the past for rapidly bringing elevated blood pressures down. At the same time, I wanted to correct the other derangements caused by the kidney failure.

I explained to Robert, and his grandmother, the necessity of keeping his BP lowered and of starting peritoneal dialysis as soon as I could make arrangements. I emphasized the urgency of these measures. They listened carefully as I went over the dialysis protocol with them.

Following additional antihypertensive medication and a forty hour dialysis, Robert's BP dropped significantly. He tolerated the treatment fairly well, in spite of the pain associated with repositioning the catheter to ensure proper drainage of the dialysis fluid. Afterwards, his headaches were less intense.

Robert remained in the hospital for another week, while we were assessing his baseline kidney function and attempting to regulate his BP. Although he was on potent blood pressure medications, I was not satisfied with the levels his BP reached, post dialysis.

I had left the dialysis catheter in place, because I wanted to perform another dialysis before discharging him, in hopes of establishing a dry weight.

Although Robert's urine volume dropped following his dialysis, about a week later it returned to his pre hospitalization output. Dropping a patient's BP, under clinical conditions such as Robert's, often compromises kidney function, at least initially, and sometimes kidney function never returns to basal levels.

We were able to collect urine and draw blood for the calculation of his creatinine clearances, shortly before discharge. They were low, but at least he did have minimal renal function. I thought Robert might be another candidate for intermittent peritoneal dialysis. I would talk to Dr. Sherman about arranging for another button implant.

Prior to Robert's discharge from the hospital, I hadn't given much thought to his hospital expenses and insurance coverage. I had not received any calls from admission, or from the administrator's office, concerning such matters. I really didn't want to discuss financial matters with him or his grandmother at that time. I felt they needed time to adjust to the fact that Robert's kidney disease was a condition for which there was no cure.

I discovered later, that Mrs. Jackson, Robert's grandmother, had a hospitalization policy through a local agency, Williams Life and Casualty. I found out, from talking with Administration, that the policy did cover Robert and his grandmother, for a small portion of the costs of hospital stays. The policy did not provide coverage for dialysis.

Before I discharged Robert from the hospital, I discussed all aspects of his condition with him and his grandmother. I explained that his kidneys were so badly damaged that they couldn't be repaired. I asked our dietitian to instruct him in food and fluid restrictions. Finally, I told him of the likely need for long-term dialytic treatments, until we could find a kidney transplant program willing to accept him. I began making enquiries around the country to locate such a program.

Robert's grandmother found it difficult to come to grips with the facts I presented. "Robert's only twenty years old, Doctor. How can this be happening? He's never had anything wrong with his health before. Are you sure there's nothing that can be done to make his kidneys better?" she pleaded.

"I wish I could give you a better answer. No, the damage has been done, not just in recent months, but over a number of years. All the studies indicate this reality. In conditions like Robert's, patients often have no signs or symptoms of kidney failure until later in life—then the blood pressure rises until it reaches a dangerous level. And, as in Robert's case, the high blood pressure causes pressure on the brain. Seizures, headaches, blurring of vision, and other symptoms may occur." As I finished talking, I said to myself, *That sounded pretty depressing.*

"Doctor V," Robert asked abruptly, "just tell me straight out, how much time do I have left?"

"Now you hush that talk, Robert," his grandmother interrupted.

"Well, wait—wait a minute, let me tell you how I see all this." I broke in. "Your kidneys can't be repaired. But peritoneal dialysis and blood pressure medications can help keep your BP down and stop the seizures. The diet you are now on may help your kidneys from deteriorating further, and in the meantime, we'll be diligently looking for somewhere to send you, for evaluation for a kidney transplant. So, we have options, peritoneal dialysis and a special type of diet." I didn't want to offer false hope, but I wanted to be as optimistic as I could.

Robert's grandmother just shook her head from side to side. She was trying to understand the significance of what she heard. "I just don't understand how all this could have happened with us not knowing anything was wrong."

Robert had listened stoically to all I had been saying. "I think ... he hesitated. "Maybe I'm beginning to see things a little clearer. I thought for a while, that the dialysis treatments were gonna make my kidneys better. I guess ... I ... just didn't want to think that they were as bad as you told me, when we first started the dialysis. But, Doc, I want to live. Maybe things won't be as bad as I first thought. I'll work with you, Doc." A slight smile flickered across his face, and then faded quickly.

I told them how sorry I was to have to lay it all out the way I did, but that I didn't know any other way. I left the hospital that night feeling down. But I told myself, good things could come from this. Robert was getting a second chance at life. We could start peritoneal dialysis as soon as the button could be implanted.

CHAPTER 13

RITA

A slender restricted diet is always dangerous in chronic diseases.
Aphorisms by Hippocrates, circa 400 B.C.E. *Translated by*
Francis Adams

I had left the hospital earlier than usual, intending to have
dinner with my family before going back to the hospital. The
phone was ringing as I opened my front door.

My wife picked up the phone, "It's the answering service."

"Tell them I'll call back in just a moment." I sank down
on the sofa.

"They said it's an emergency. You'll need to talk with
them now." She handed me the phone.

"Doctor, you have a patient in the Emergency Room. I'll
connect you," Doris, at the switchboard, informed me.

"Doctor V, your patient, Rita Kimble was brought in by
Floyd County ambulance, about ten minutes ago. She's in a
good bit of respiratory distress and very apprehensive. Dr.
Amos Job, the Intern on Medicine, is with her now," Reba
Beckworth, the ER charge nurse reported.

Fifteen minutes later, I was back at University's ER.
Mrs. Kimble was in pulmonary edema, a severe circulatory
congestive state. Dr. Job had put light tourniquets on all

extremities. She was being administered nasal oxygen, and had been given an intravenous injection of Sodium Bicarbonate. Also, she received a small dose of Morphine, which helped relieve her anxiety from almost drowning in her bodily fluids.

Leaning over her bedside railing, I touched her hand lightly. She was propped upright and apparently breathing somewhat better than on admission. I told her we were going to do peritoneal dialysis, "… just like that first time, when Dr. Billingsley asked me to see you."

She nodded her head. I knew she understood.

I started the dialysis in the ER. The procedure was more difficult than usual. She could not lie flat in the bed because of her congestion. Smaller amounts of dialysis fluids had to be instilled at first, to minimize pressure on her diaphragm, and avoid compromising her breathing.

Within about ten rapid exchanges, her condition improved enough that she could be moved to Barrett 2 — the designated dialysis room. I stayed with Mrs. Kimble until her blood work improved and her labored breathing had abated. Initially, her electrocardiogram reflected her elevated serum potassium level, which was 7.5 meq/l. After the IV bicarbonate and with dialysis, it dropped to normal over the next several hours.

Although there were no clearances to go by, Mrs. Kimble's BUN and serum creatinine were essentially the same as on her last visit to my office, as best I recalled. However, she was in a moderately acidotic state, in spite of the alkalizing (Shohls) solution she'd been taking.

The dialysis continued through the night. I left around midnight, telling her I'd be back early in the morning. Again, she nodded her head and said, "You go on home, Doc, and get yourself some rest."

When I arrived for rounds the next morning, Mrs. Kimble apologized for "them havin' to call you back to the hospital last night. But I remembered that you did say for me to come to Augusta, if I had any more problems. So, here I am," she smiled.

Before Mrs. Kimble's discharge, I asked Dr. Jim Dickson, a Cardiologist and close friend, if he would see her in consultation. I explained that she had no hospitalization insurance and would not be able to pay for his services. But I knew when Jim learned of her dire circumstances, he would have no hesitation in seeing her. He was that kind of doctor. After he had seen Mrs. Kimble and reviewed her clinical course, Jim called me at my office.

"George," he said. "Mrs. Kimble does have an enlarged heart, but I believe it's likely that the dysrhythmia, related to her hyperkalemia, caused her pulmonary edema last night. Her initial cardiogram, before she was administered bicarb, showed a slow junctional rhythm. This converted to a regular sinus shortly afterwards, and she obviously responded dramatically to dialysis and the correction of her acidosis. I did talk to her about the critical need for her to stay on her diet—that it was truly a matter of life and death. I ordered some cardiac enzymes, which I'll check on before she leaves the hospital. I'd be glad to see her again if she gets into more trouble in the future."

I thanked Jim for his looking in on Mrs. Kimble, and for his thoughts on her condition. The next afternoon, she was back to her usual self, and I dismissed her. Her cardiac enzymes were normal. I told her to call my office for an appointment in two days.

This was the second time in recent months, that Mrs. Kimble's potassium level proved to be dangerously high, in spite of the serious attention, I knew, she gave to her diet.

Since Mrs. Kimble's admission to the hospital was an emergency, I'd had no trouble admitting her. But I knew that starting her on regular hospital dialysis treatments was not an option. University administration had let me know they were not interested in sponsoring other non-insured patients for regular dialysis treatments.

I WAS EVALUATING more and more patients with chronic kidney failure. Because treatment options for that condition were limited, I spent much time in the Medical College of Georgia's library, searching the *Index Medicus* — an extensive listing of thousands of medical journals — for any new management regimens for these patients.

Other groups were confirming the early experiences of the Italian physicians, Sergio Giovannetti and Carmelo Giordano, with very low protein diets. Some patients were living for extended periods, many months to several years, on modifications of the original diet alone. Many of them were living normal lives, without uremic symptoms. If they adhered to these diets, they tended to be free of nausea and vomiting, had good appetites, and felt good. Mrs. Kimble certainly fit that characterization.

However, an increasing number of patients, on these very low protein diets, were dying suddenly. Terminally, they had some of the same findings (high serum potassium and acidosis) as Mrs. Kimble when she was recently hospitalized and dialyzed. I was concerned that her present regimen might not be the best. Mrs. Kimble needed to be on a regularly scheduled dialysis treatment program. I was determined to find a way to dialyze her with the frequency she needed.

CHAPTER 14

OUTPATIENT DIALYSIS

"The World's first outpatient dialysis center, the Seattle Artificial Kidney Center, was established in 1962." *American J. Nephrol. 1999; 19(2) abstract; Blagg, C.R*

Mrs. Kimble kept her appointment. Her friend, Helen, again had driven her to town. She said, "I'm feelin' 'bout as good as I was 'fore I got sick last week, Doc, 'cept for jist a little bit of nausea, on occasion, that's all."

After I had checked her over briefly, I said, "Mrs. Kimble, I've become more and more concerned that ... I know you're staying on your diet. I know you know how important that is—"

"Doc," she interrupted. "There were times 'fore this last attack I had, that I wasn't stickin' as close to my diet as I should. But after that time when I went to Floyd County Hospital, I made a promise to myself that I wasn't gonna let my likes for certain foods put me in that shape again. So, this last spell, I don't know how it happened. I've been on my diet, I'd say 'bout a hundred percent."

"Yes, and I believe you. Which brings me to what I want to talk to you about. You see, this strict diet you've been on has some drawbacks. Sometimes it hides the symptoms of uremia. You know, the fatigue, nausea, and lack of appetite you were experiencing when I first saw you? This may be the reason you're not having uremic symptoms while you stay strictly on your diet. The diet keeps them from returning. But, in spite of everything you're doing right, your kidneys are not getting any better. The diet and fluid restriction are not making the kidneys heal. At best, they're hiding some of the usual symptoms of uremia."

"You mean, Doc, we're gonna have to change my diet?"

"No, I don't want to change your diet. But I feel it's time to set up a regularly scheduled time for you to be dialyzed. Dialyzing just when you get into trouble is too dangerous. The diet alone is, frankly, just not enough. Like I said, I don't want to change your diet, I just want to add dialysis to your treatment program—diet plus dialysis. The last clearances we had showed that your kidney function was lower than ever. It's just too dangerous to continue trying to manage your kidney condition with diet alone."

"Doc, you think the hospital'll let me come in, right regular like?"

"Well, there's the hitch. I've been doing a lot of thinking about that. Suppose you didn't have to be in the hospital for your dialysis treatments?"

"How'd that work, Doc.?"

"Mrs. Kimble, you tolerate the dialysis procedure so well, I believe we should be able to dialyze you somewhere other than in a hospital. If my office had one more exam room, we could use that space. We could dialyze you there, but we don't have the space. We need to find a room—a location—somewhere that would be safe. And I've come to the conclusion that a motel might just be that suitable place."

Mrs. Kimble seemed totally nonplussed by my suggestion: dialysis out of the hospital—in a motel? Or, by the fact that now she would have to be on a regular schedule for dialysis. "Well, if that's what you think we should do, then let's get at it. But you'll have to give me a few days to get things straight at home. When should I come back?"

I knew that setting regular times for dialysis treatments was going to create problems — she would need to depend on her friend, Helen, for transportation to and from Augusta, as their own truck was not in a drivable condition. Besides, she told me she had no money to buy gas. She was going to have to be sure that dialysis didn't keep her from being home when her two youngest children returned from school. She knew her husband wouldn't be able to manage the kids and house by himself.

I said, "I think we'll be able to help you make the sort of arrangements necessary for the dialysis treatment to take place."

I was sure that University Hospital would not agree to having Mrs. Kimble on a chronic in-house dialysis program. But Mrs. Kimble needed to be on a chronic dialysis program — somewhere. Also, I had confidence that the dialysis team I'd been working with in the hospital was capable of managing peritoneal dialysis safely in an outpatient facility.

I told her I would find a proper facility for dialysis and would give her six or seven days before starting regularly scheduled treatments. I hoped that a thirty-six to forty hour treatment about every ten days would suffice.

I DIDN'T HEAR from Mrs. Kimble again until the night before she was to have her first outpatient dialysis. She called my office wanting to know where she was to go for the treatment. I told her I had decided on the University Motel, near my office on Central Avenue, and across the street from University Hospital. She was to come to my office around two o'clock, and we would take her to the motel.

The motel was new and usually never filled. I had called the middle of the week and booked a room, for two nights, Friday and Saturday. I requested a room on the ground floor. I wanted to be able to visit as quickly as possible if I was needed for an emergency. And if, for whatever reason, dialysis fluids were spilled, there would be no guests below to get drenched.

Right on time the next day, Mrs. Kimble and her friend Helen arrived at my office.

"How has your week been?" I asked.

"Everythin' about the same 'cept for that same little bit'a nausea I've been havin' every now an' then, Doc. How you been doin'?"

"Fine," I replied, smiling.

Janet drove the two of them to the motel and checked in without incident. About an hour later, I brought over the dialysis supplies and an IV stand. We set up for the procedure. Previously, I had arranged for Sally McKinnon and Jean Phillips, two of the nurses who were skilled in running peritoneal dialysis in the hospital, to help with this outpatient treatment.

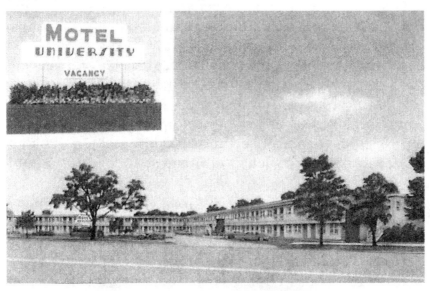

Old postcard of University Motel

There were two single beds in the room. Mrs. Kimble stretched out on the one nearest the door. We warmed the bottles of dialysis solutions to body temperature in the bathtub.

I started the dialysis on Mrs. Kimble as I had previously. When I felt comfortable that they could proceed successfully and safely without me, I left to see patients in the hospital. I told Mrs. Kimble and Ms. McKinnon I'd be back shortly.

When I returned, several hours later, everything was going smoothly. Mrs. Kimble had been sleeping off and on. Drainage of the dialysis solutions in and out was excellent. Ms. McKinnon assured me that she would be able to manage without me being present.

Mrs. Kimble reached out for Sally's hand, "Don't you worry about us, Doc." She winked, "I trust this girl with my life."

I went home in the early morning hours, but didn't sleep well. I kept waking up and worrying about my patient. I was back in the motel at six A.M., just as the shift was changing.

Ms. McKinnon was giving report to Ms. Phillips, who would take the next twelve-hour shift. Ms. McKinnon, then, would return for the final shift.

"How did the night go?" I asked Mrs. Kimble.

"Fine. All the nausea's gone and I got my appetite back." She smiled happily, eating a doughnut her "night nurse" had provided.

This outpatient dialysis had gone exceptionally well. Mrs. Kimble slept most of the night. There had been no complications.

At the time, I thought this arrangement—motel outpatient peritoneal dialysis—might be a treatment option for other patients. The room cost eight dollars a night. I engaged Sally McKinnon and Jean Phillips at the usual private duty nurse rate of ten dollars. I had added two more dollars to account for the extra long shift.

So, basic costs for a 36-hour dialysis in a motel "clinic" would be less than fifty dollars, not counting my fees— which for patients like Mrs. Kimble, I was omitting—and miscellaneous items. And, if the dialysis suppliers continued to donate the supplies and equipment ... then maybe I would be able to increase the frequency of dialytic treatments for other under-dialyzed patients. Could motel dialysis clinics be a wave of the future?

We started the dialysis treatment at seven o'clock P.M., Friday, and finished at seven A.M., Sunday. Mrs. Kimble's friend, Helen, came by at eight to take her home.

Mrs. Kimble received her second motel dialysis two weeks later. Again, the procedure went well technically, and Mrs. Kimble tolerated it with her usual good patient demeanor. But, I thought, if we were to be able to continue dialyzing in University Motel, I should let the management know what we were doing. They might begin to have suspicions that some sort of shenanigans were going on. The same group of people coming every two weeks to the same requested room. Of course, they might have justified objections to our using their motel for a clinic. *They surely might*, I thought. Then again, maybe once they understood the dire circumstances of some patients with chronic kidney failure, they would be willing to aid us in our endeavors. Maybe they would offer us a discounted rate!

MRS. KIMBLE'S 24-hour urine volumes were declining along with her creatinine clearances. She phoned my office on a Wednesday before the weekend of her next planned outpatient dialysis, and left a message with my receptionist that she "wasn't feeling good." She told her she was getting dizzy whenever she stood too quickly. Janet relayed the message to me as I was making rounds at University.

I called the Kimble's home and daughter Evelyn answered. She had come over, after talking with her mother earlier, to check on her. Evelyn said her mother looked "very pale and was acting nervous-like, rubbing her hands together like she's cold, when I got here. But now she's out like a light. I can't get her to respond to me. Her hands are like ice and she's not breathing right, Doc. I'm afraid she's leaving us. What should I do?" Evelyn's voice was high pitched, but calm.

I told her to call the ambulance service, and get her to University ER fast as they could. I would meet them there.

I arrived in the ER before the ambulance. About fifteen minutes later, it drove up with it's lights blinking and siren blasting. Tom Griffin, the driver and a friend for many years, came over quickly to where I was waiting on the ER receiving platform.

Tom owned the local Griffin Funeral Home and had been working for the ambulance service for over twenty years. He was very competent in managing emergency situations and I trusted his clinical skills. "Doc," he said, shaking his head, "she's already gone. She had no vital signs when we first checked her out in the house. We did what we could, but we got no response with resuscitation. We continued it all the way here. The family was following us, Evelyn, her brother and sisters — even Mr. Kimble. They're taking it right hard. They're in the waiting room."

I went over to the stretcher on which Mrs. Kimble was lying. I had the ambulance attendant remove the mask and the oral airway. I put my stethoscope on her chest and listened. It was just a formality. I made my way slowly to the waiting room.

The Kimbles: Luke, Evelyn, Herbert, and the two youngest, Timmy and Sarah, were huddled around a small table. They were very quiet. Timmy and Sarah were holding hands. Tears streaked their faces. The others were stoic. I put my hand out to touch Herbert's shoulder. "She didn't make it. I think y'all know." The grownups came over to me and said they *did* know, even before the ambulance arrived. "She tried to do everythin' she was supposed to do and it never seemed enough," Luke offered. "Doctor," Mr. Kimble managed to say, "we know you did all you could and we're grateful. She suffered so much. She's with her Lord now."

I was beyond sad. Emotionally drained, and angry. We knew how and should have done better.

CHAPTER 15

JIMMY

"We now regard isolated jejunal loop dialysis as an efficient method of home dialysis in properly selected patients." **Isolated Small Bowel Dialysis in 23 Patients. J.E. Clark et al Transactions American Society Artificial Internal Organs Vol. XI 1965**

It was Friday morning. I was on call for my group, and making rounds at University, when the hospital switchboard operator paged me. She had Nettie Wells, Jimmy Wells' sister, on the line.

"Doc, Jimmy's not doing well." Her voice was high pitched and she was speaking fast. "He doesn't plan to come in for his regular dialysis today. He's got off his diet in a big way. He's gained, probably, I'd say, at least ten pounds over the last week. I don't know exactly how much, 'cause he won't let me weigh 'im. He's really havin' trouble breathin'. And you already know how depressed he is, Doc. He didn't want me to call you, but I think you better see him in the ER, right away. I'm gonna try to make him go. Hold on a minute … hold on … he wants to talk to you."

WHEN JIMMY CAME IN for his dialysis two weeks ago, I couldn't slide the skin over the button and insert the catheter without it kinking. I'd been having trouble with the insertion over the last month, but now it had become impossible to position it and administer the dialysate effectively. I felt I couldn't rely on the button any more. And I knew this was going to be a big problem for Jimmy.

"DOC, I JUST DON'T WANT to dialyze any more. It's not worth it to me. I could just barely tolerate the dialysis with the button, and now, since it can't be used ... I know, I need dialyzing, but—"

"Jimmy," I interrupted. "Jimmy, wait a minute. You remember, a couple of weeks ago, when you came in for your dialysis, I said I was looking into an alternative method of dialyzing, and that it might be something that you should consider? Well, I think now is the time to seriously consider it.

"This is a different kind of dialysis; not a different kind of peritoneal dialysis, but something totally different. I'll explain it to you after you come in to the hospital. You're fed up with peritoneals. I know, I understand. But this other treatment option, I want you to think about ... I want to go over it in detail with you, in person, not over the phone. You still need dialyzing just to remove fluid, if for no other reason. I want you to, at least, hear about this other treatment. Will you do that? Just give me a chance to talk with you about it. Okay?"

Except for labored breathing, there was silence on the other end of the line. I waited. I didn't plead further. I waited. Then, in a flat monotone, "Okay, Doc, I'll come. I'll have ... I'll have my dialysis, and listen to what you have to say. I'm not sayin' I'll do it—this new treatment you're talkin' about—I'm just sayin' I'll listen."

Several months ago, I had begun rereading the articles, and reprints I had collected on Intestinal Dialysis. Jimmy's peritoneals were keeping him alive, but affording him little respite from his uremia. Being as depressed as he was, he could not visualize any realistic way out of his unacceptable existence. His quality of life was zero on a scale of ten. I knew he was very close to giving up.

The artificial kidney was not an option for him. There were no programs set up for long-term hemo or peritoneal dialysis in the Central Savannah River Area (CSRA). Medical centers around the country had either not begun such programs, or were overwhelmed with their own groups of patients. As such, they had no interest in, or capabilities of, accepting patients not already known to them.

THE CONCEPT of using the intestines for dialysis in treating renal failure was not new. Still, in spite of years of interest and research on the usefulness of perfusion of the intestines for kidney failure, intestinal dialysis had not established itself in clinical medicine. I had considered it to be, at best, an adjunct treatment, along with hemo or peritoneal dialysis in special clinical circumstances. Most studies showed the procedure was very effective in removing excess fluid, but not in controlling uremia in the long term.

However, J.E. Clark and Associates recently reported, in the *Transactions of the American Society of Artificial Internal Organs* (ASAIO), their experiences treating twenty-three patients with chronic renal failure by intestinal dialysis. They made a strong case for using intestinal dialysis alone, as a viable alternative to hemo and peritoneal dialysis in carefully selected patients.

Although many of their patients died early on, four were still living at the time of the report. One, with essentially no kidney function, had been on intestinal dialysis for twenty-six months. She had no loss of appetite, no nausea, no vomiting— no uremic symptoms. They reported that this housewife was living a normal life, in spite of being essentially anephric— without kidney function. The three other patients, all with very minimal kidney function, also were free of uremic symptoms. They all started their intestinal dialyses in the hospital, but the four of them now were doing their own treatments at home, with only the aid of family members.

Could this be the answer for Jimmy? Would he tolerate this better than he had been tolerating peritoneal dialysis? I didn't dwell on the question. I focused on the possibility that this just might work for Jimmy. I was grasping for straws. At the same time, I thought this might be a stopgap measure, viable enough to offer him a temporary reprieve from the misery he was suffering. And maybe, just maybe, buy him enough time to get that elusive transplant.

I met Jimmy and Nettie in the ER shortly after noon. A critical bed shortage in the Augusta area had developed in the last several years. The room that had been set aside for dialysis was, more and more frequently, used for general medical beds. Jimmy was told he'd have to wait, until one or both of the patients in that room were discharged or moved to another room, before he could reclaim it for his dialysis. Fortunately, his condition was not as critical as I had expected. He was having some trouble breathing, but was stable enough to wait, without much discomfort, while the room was being readied for dialysis.

I didn't try to use the button because of my last failed encounter with it. I gave him a mild sedative, and started the dialysis the way I had before the button was implanted. Jimmy complained very little. He accepted the necessity of the procedure and, seemingly, resigned himself to it. Some three liters of fluid were removed during the next twenty-four hours.

I made no attempt to talk with Jimmy during his dialysis. He was in no mood to talk with me either. He was quiet during the treatment and slept much of the time. I terminated the dialysis after thirty-six hours. His blood work was now in an acceptable range. Removing the excess fluid was the main goal at this time.

Afterward, with Nettie watching, I pulled up a chair next to Jimmy's bed. He was asleep, but quickly woke when I spoke to him.

"I feel better now, Doc. Guess I didn't realize how much all that extra fluid was affectin' me." He sounded more energized.

"Well, do you feel up to listening to what I have to tell you about this different form of dialysis?"

"Yeah, I do. I wanna hear about it. I'm even gettin' a little hope it might work. And I don't even know a thing about it yet. Doc, you know ... I ... I appreciate all you, and Nettie, are doing for me. I don't want to be a difficult patient. I shouldn't get the feelings I do about not wantin' to live the way I've been livin' — but I do. I can't seem to help it."

"Jimmy, you're not a difficult patient. What's difficult is you having to put up with these treatments."

At that moment, I resented chronic kidney disease. I resented the fact that Jimmy had to suffer its effects. I resented that there were no dialysis machines available for him. I resented that there were no kidney transplant centers ready to take him. I resented that I couldn't help Jimmy overcome all the bad things that were happening to him.

I was doing everything I could. I wanted desperately for him to make it. If he could only hang on for a few more months, maybe — just maybe — he could get to Richmond for the transplant.

"The treatment I'm talking about is called 'intestinal dialysis,'" I said. "It would require surgery. A small loop of intestine is separated from the main body of the intestines. This loop, with its blood supply intact, remains within your abdominal cavity. Each end of the loop is brought to the inner surface of your abdominal wall where two openings are made in the skin and connected to the loops. So there would be two outside openings in your belly wall. When not in use these openings would be covered with a bandage.

"A dialyzing solution would be instilled in one opening and drained through the other opening. As the solution moves through the intestinal segment it washes out intestinal fluid along with toxic products that have accumulated in your body resulting from your kidney failure. The solutions would be allowed to flow by gravity and the rate of flow controlled by a screw clamp, just as when you receive IV fluids."

I told him that I had already talked with Dr. Sherman about the surgical procedure. "Dr. Sherman has reviewed the surgical protocol, and has advised me that he could do the surgery, which shouldn't take very long, as soon as you're scheduled.

"Jimmy, we would start the treatments in the hospital. But, the good part is you'll be able to continue them at home, and on your own schedule. Some of the patients, who have had this type of dialysis, take the treatments while they sleep."

"Doc, what will takin' a part of my intestines out do to me, I mean, how about my bowel movements, and things like that?"

"Well, as soon as the small segment is removed, the intestine is immediately hooked back up. You have over 20 feet of small intestine. Only about 5 feet are removed, so, you should have no problem with your digestion. Your intestinal tract should function as well as it did before surgery."

"You're tellin' me now, that with this new treatment, there won't be puncturin' my belly with needles or catheters, stickin' tubes in my belly, or anythin' like that?"

"Right, the only tubes will be two soft catheters, one placed in each intestinal opening. No pain with this procedure. They will only be in place, when the fluids are dripping in. After the dialysis is finished, you will use a small patch much like a large band-aid to cover the openings. You and Nettie will be shown how to prepare the solutions, how much water, glucose, salt, bicarbonate and whatever else needs to be added, depending on your blood chemistries."

I explained to Jimmy and Nettie that this procedure had been around for a number of years. I told them that some of the earlier reports had been successful, but some of the later studies were not as promising. I went on to say, that I was encouraged by the latest reports of Drs. James Clark and his associates, in Philadelphia at the Jefferson Medical College. I told them about their four patients who were treating themselves at home. All four had less kidney function than

Jimmy; and one had practically none. I told them she had been on intestinal dialysis for over two years, and was living a normal life, without any of the symptoms of uremia.

I wanted Jimmy to be convinced that this was something he wanted to try. I wanted him to know all that he could know about the treatment. He seemed encouraged to learn about a dialysis modality that he might be able to live with.

"I'll go for it Doc," he said. "Don't you agree, Nettie?"

"Oh, yes, I do. When can we start, Doc?"

"I'll give Dr. Sherman a call in the A.M. and see when he can schedule surgery."

Jimmy's surgery lasted a little under two hours and was without complications. He had a smile on his face when I met him in the recovery room, after he had awoke from the anesthesia.

"We will start the treatment tomorrow," I said. "First, we need two plastic carboys—tanks—large enough for the six liters of dialysis solution. I've already located a warehouse that has that exact size. The pharmacy will prepare the solutions, after I write prescriptions for the amounts of glucose and salts needed."

"Nettie told me she has arranged to be off for the next three days. I don't think she will need all that time, really, to learn the procedure. It's relatively straight forward: mix the glucose and other ingredients in plain tap water, warmed to body temperature in the carboys, hook up the lines for inflow and output, insert them into the Foley catheters that have been placed in the two intestinal openings, and adjust the solution to run in over six hours."

Jimmy remained hospitalized for the next two days. Both he and Nettie learned the technique of intestinal dialysis quickly. They both were optimistic about this new treatment.

While in the hospital, Jimmy underwent two dialyses. One was done during the night while he slept, and it went smoothly. The plan at home was to do the treatments nightly five days in a row, then no treatments for two days. Then repeat the cycle. Arrangements were made for the hospital pharmacy to supply enough ingredients for the dialysate to last two weeks. The carboys went home with the Wells.

"Doc," Jimmy said as he was leaving the hospital. "When can I get rid of this button? I don't expect to ever need it again!"

I told him I'd get in touch with Dr. Sherman. "The two of you can set a time for that, whenever y'all can get together."

CHAPTER 16

ROBERT

"Both chronic dialysis and transplantation ... are considered clinical experiments rather than established modes of treatment ...." **Renal Failure Part 2; Norman Levinsky; Management of Chronic NEJM. 271; 1964**

Robert had now been undergoing peritoneal dialysis for the last three months. Initially, we used the button and he dialyzed every three weeks. With dialysis and antihypertensives, he'd had no more seizures. His kidney function had improved some, but he still required dialysis when his uremic symptoms recurred.

His hospitalizations were partially covered by the small insurance policy his grandmother owned. For the first several hospitalizations, University had no objections to Robert being admitted. However, during his fourth admission, Mr. Higgans asked me to stop by his office for a chat. He asked how long Robert would need peritoneal dialysis. I told him, I wish I knew the answer to that.

"Well," Mr. Higgans began. "We have a small problem. That little insurance policy of Mrs. Jackson pays for less than half of the cost of a hospital room. It pays nothing for the dialysis supplies, equipment, and the extra nurses needed for the procedure."

"Mr. Higgans," I replied. "I believe I can make the same arrangements for Robert that I was able to make for Jimmy Wells. I haven't spoken to Bill Sessions at Baxter/Travenol about this, but I think he would be willing to provide the supplies and equipment necessary for continuing the dialyses. Also, I can have my nurse more readily available to help with the dialysis."

"Doctor, I'm afraid there's a little more to this than just the expenses of long term dialysis. Some on the Executive Committee have questioned the propriety of the University Hospital becoming a facility for chronic dialysis. Some have even questioned the ethics of keeping patients alive with a treatment that some feel is still experimental."

"Well, that does put this in a different light." I was a little perplexed. "I don't envision University Hospital evolving into a chronic dialysis facility. I know some still consider dialysis for chronic renal failure to be experimental. On the other hand, peritoneal dialysis has been utilized successfully as a treatment option for many patients with CRD over the last few years in a number of locales in the US, and in other countries."

"Yes, I too am aware of that. But these treatments are taking place in medical centers, not in community hospitals," Mr. Higgans replied. "And, they are subsidized by governmental or other institutional grants, not by community hospitals."

"You're right, of course," I conceded. "But please understand, starting a chronic dialysis center at University is not something I'm interested in. I really just want to give this one particular patient, this one young man who deserves a chance to live, an opportunity to survive long enough to receive a kidney transplant. As far as the ethical issue is concerned, I'll stick with my approach to treating patients with chronic renal failure. As long as I know how to perform peritoneal dialysis, and companies continue making the equipment and supplies for dialysis, I'll continue looking for a place to dialyze. In my opinion it would be unethical to do otherwise. Of course, that's just my opinion. Others are certainly entitled to theirs." I didn't want this to come off as confrontational, but I wanted Higgans to see where I stood.

I needed his support if Robert was to continue in-hospital dialysis. I told him that Robert's grandmother's church was planning a benefit for her grandson sometime within the next month.

"I don't know how much money this will raise, but surely, whatever amount is raised, will help in defraying some of the hospital's shortfall." I wasn't sure how administration would react to this information, but I had hopes. Anyway, Robert was in the hospital now, and being dialyzed, as we talked.

Between dialyses, Robert was staying relatively free of uremic symptoms. He was receiving peritoneal dialysis on an as needed basis—usually every three weeks. His headaches and blurred vision were gone. His blood pressure was better controlled, and in fact, his creatinine clearances had shown a small but definite improvement. His kidneys were actually working better.

CHAPTER 17

THE ARTIFICIAL KIDNEY

"Saving lives is serious business and members of the Women's Board of University Hospital ... The latest evidence of the Board's relentless efforts to aid University Hospital is its decision to purchase an artificial kidney to be used for hospital patients." **Augusta Chronicle, October 24, 1965**

In the fall of 1965, the Women's Board of University Hospital invited me to speak to them about the artificial kidney. That year, as their contribution to patient care, they planned to purchase a dialysis machine for the hospital. Proceeds from an "Old South Ball" they were hosting later in the year, would go to buying the machine. They estimated the cost to be around $2000.

I gave them a short history of hemodialysis—using an artificial kidney—and an overview of the technique of dialysis. I pointed out this dialysis machine would likely be used only for patients with acute problems; that is, patients who, ordinarily would be expected to recover from a kidney injury or condition, or for treating patients with drug overdoses or poisons—not for patients who needed the long term support of an artificial kidney in order to live.

Some of the ladies at the talk were surprised to learn that the University Hospital, after acquiring an artificial kidney, would not be using it to extend the lives of all patients dying from kidney failure. I explained that recently some centers in this country, and overseas had started such programs for chronic kidney failure. Moreover, that these programs were generally supported by academic medical centers or governmental institutions. Their success depended on the continued financial support and commitments from groups of professionals dedicated to long-term goals.

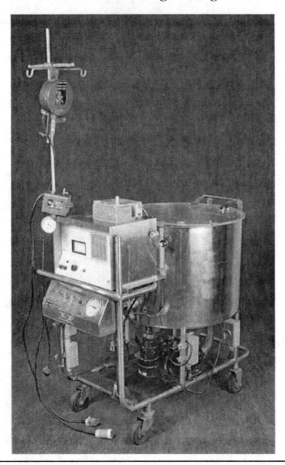

Travenol dialysis machine model U200A, same as 'artificial kidney' purchased by Women's Board University Hospital.

HEMODIALYSIS REQUIRES access to a patient's circulation. In the early years, this necessitated exposing an artery and a vein, via a surgical cutdown. Needles were placed in the vessels, and when the dialysis was completed the needles were, ordinarily, removed. Frequently, this procedure resulted in the loss of one or both vessels. Sometimes, in patients undergoing acute dialyses, needles in an artery and a vein were left in place for several days; but in patients requiring repeated dialyses, over months or longer, leaving the needles in place was not feasible.

If hemodialysis was to become a practical technique for treating patients with chronic kidney failure, a permanent access to the circulation was a necessity. Belding Scribner's group, in Seattle, designed such an access. They began using their Teflon Silastic shunt for chronic kidney failure in the early 1960s. Their shunt consisted of flexible tubing, with Teflon tips, for insertion into vessels near the wrist. One went into an artery and the other into a nearby vein. Other similar shunt devices soon appeared.

Not infrequently, shunts like these clotted, became infected, malfunctioned, or totally failed after five or six months — or sooner. In the early years of chronic hemodialysis, the coils for the dialysis machines were large and required the use of blood for priming the lines for each dialysis. At first, the hospital pharmacy prepared the ingredients for the dialysis solutions according to prescriptions written by the physicians in charge of the dialysis. All these issues added to the complexity and cost of hemodialysis.

Later, after the Cimino/Brescia Arterial Venous fistula became the standard for vascular access for hemodialysis, and Medicare covered essentially all patients with chronic renal failure, Hemodialysis established itself over peritoneal dialysis as the preferable mode of treatment for end stage renal disease.

IN 1965, I was still wedded to the concept of peritoneal dialysis, rather than hemodialysis, as the more practical method for managing chronic kidney failure—a procedure both simple and inexpensive. Having access to hemodialysis would be a boon for treating patients with acute conditions.

Though both hemo and peritoneal dialysis perform basically the same functions, when it comes to relieving the symptoms of uremia and removing toxic products from the body, hemodialysis is a more efficient method. Having an artificial kidney, when it came to treating patients with poisons, drug overdoses, and acute kidney failure, would give UH a state of the art treatment modality. However, to use hemodialysis for the regular treatment of patients with chronic progressive renal failure in a city/county hospital like University was, to my way of thinking at the time, unfeasible.

CHAPTER 18

THE BUTTON - AGAIN

It has been said that the height of futility is to do the same thing over and over and expect different results. **Anon**

Since beginning my practice in Augusta in 1963, I had used peritoneal dialysis for patients with acute kidney failure and with drug overdoses, as well as for those with chronic kidney failure, like Rita Kimble, Jimmy Wells, and now, Robert Jackson.

Then, I didn't see a need for an artificial kidney in the management of patients with chronic kidney failure. Peritoneal dialysis, much simpler and less expensive, would suffice. But my approach to managing chronic progressive renal failure was evolving. If a patient needed dialysis every three to four weeks, the method was workable. However, more frequent dialysis was required for those with very little renal function. For them, the intermittent puncture technique was proving to be impractical. Soon, it became obvious to me, as well as others in the dialysis community, that three to four weeks between dialyses was too long an interval for most patients. Intermittent puncture of the peritoneal membrane every week, or more frequently, was not a treatment procedure many patients would tolerate.

The button I was using should eliminate that obstacle of puncturing the peritoneal membrane. If I could only get it to function properly. In the meantime, indwelling catheters for peritoneal dialysis came into clinical practice. Several other modifications of a button also survived for a short time.

Although I arranged for Robert Jackson to have the button implanted and had already begun using it for dialysis, after three very difficult dialyses, I accepted the fact that the procedure was not working as it should. As with Jimmy Well's dialyses, the angle between the catheter and the button remained too acute and the catheter invariably kinked. I arranged to have his button removed.

ROBERT'S CLEARANCES had improved enough that he could tolerate a three-week interval between dialyses, and the intermittent puncture technique would meet his needs. I didn't want to implant a permanent peritoneal catheter. I was concerned, that instead of simplifying peritoneal dialysis, the surgical implantation of a permanent catheter created a more complex situation. Also, I was unsure how effective this catheter would turn out to be. Would the dialysis solution drain in and out readily? If not, would I have to implant another catheter, along with additional surgery? In addition, I was concerned about the indwelling catheter becoming infected with ensuing peritonitis. All in all, it was a complexity I wasn't interested in pursuing.

Over the next several months, I was referred three new patients with chronic renal disease. Each of them was in a different stage of kidney failure. After I evaluated and determined that two of them, Julia Kanovich and Howard Dubinion, were uremic and in need of dialysis, I decided to try my buttons again. I still wanted — hoped — peritoneal dialysis to be the practical, temporary, therapeutic option for patients with chronic renal failure, until the definitive treatment, kidney transplantation, could be performed.

The buttons I used for Jimmy Wells and Robert Jackson, had been implanted in the midline of the abdomen wall, three to four centimeters below the umbilicus. I had an idea that implanting them in another location might afford me the ability to better align the peritoneal catheter with the button. I was hoping that the skin in the right and left lower quadrants of the abdomen would stretch more easily, and the angle of the catheter through the skin and into the button would be less acute, thereby allowing a freer flow of dialysate.

I dialyzed each of these patients twice, using this different button site. Changing its place in the abdominal wall did not correct the problem. The catheter continued to kink. The angle was still too acute. I ended up having the buttons removed from both patients and returned to using intermittent puncture, whenever they needed dialysis.

Both of these patients had enough kidney reserve to tolerate three to four week intervals between dialyses. On this regimen, each remained free of uremic symptoms for many months. Fortunately, both patients had some hospitalization insurance. Their policies afforded them relatively easy access to hospitalization. I continued to receive dialysis supplies, for use in the hospital, from several of the medical supply companies. Both of these advantages allowed these two patients to continue in house dialysis on an as needed basis.

Julia Kanovich was forty-seven, and Howard Dubinion, fifty-six. Because of their ages—forty to forty-five, were the cut off ages—and because they had no potential, related, donors, they were not candidates for kidney transplants.

Today, as I write this story, and try to recall my thinking then, I ask myself what was my end game? Why was I willing to start intermittent peritoneal dialysis on these patients when there were no transplant or dialysis programs available to accept them?

My thinking was that by changing the locations of the buttons in the abdominal wall, peritoneal dialysis could continue to be used as a simple and effective treatment modality for chronic kidney failure; until transplant programs relaxed their criteria for acceptance, and older patients became eligible for the transplant. Or until some other more effective mode of therapy became available. When it became obvious that my button dialysis was not going to work, I had the buttons removed and never tried them again.

I knew that by doing nothing, these patients' fates were sealed. With their degree of kidney dysfunction, without dialysis support or a transplant, their life expectancy was likely limited to months. In spite of the inadequacy of their treatment programs, I felt morally and ethically committed to continue their dialyses.

With the removal of the last button—from Julia Kanovich—I no longer focused strictly on peritoneal dialysis as the only dialytic treatment modality for chronic renal failure. My button dialysis system, with its design flaws, wasn't going to work. I wanted nothing to do with the potential complications of dialyzing through an implanted dialysis catheter. Intermittent puncture peritoneal dialysis only worked for a few selected patients.

The Scribner shunt had been in clinical practice long enough to have become the accepted method for accessing blood vessels for hemodialysis. More and more centers were offering hemodialysis for chronic renal failure.

I needed to find a way of incorporating hemodialysis into my treatment protocol for patients needing dialysis. Dr. Merrill's group in Boston, Belding Scribner's in Seattle, and Stanley Shaldon's in London, had begun regular hemodialysis programs for chronic renal failure.

Maybe hemodialysis was beginning to be accepted as mainstream treatment for chronic progressive renal failure. University Hospital did have a dialysis machine. It sat idle much of the time on the second floor of the Barrett wing. It was the same type of dialysis machine some clinics already were using for the regular treatment of chronic kidney failure. But still, University Hospital was not the location to begin a chronic dialysis program. I would have to find another alternative. At that time, I did not know what that would be.

CHAPTER 19

JIMMY

> *"I am not eager, bold, nor strong,*
> *All that is past;*
> *I am ready not to do,*
> *At last, at last."*
> *from:*
> **REST a poem by Mary Woolsey Howland**

Jimmy Wells had been dialyzing at home, via his small intestine, for the last three months. His weight fluctuations were much less than when he was on peritoneal dialysis. His uremia was better controlled, though he was still nauseous from time to time. He had occasional episodes of "nervousness," but admitted that; overall, he was a "little better off" than prior to beginning treatments.

He was still dialyzing five days a week and for the most part was able to take the treatment during his bedtime hours. His blood pressure was better controlled and he had arrived at a weight I considered close to dry.

I was seeing him in the office once every six weeks now. There was no word from any of the transplant centers I had contacted. His intestinal loop was functioning satisfactorily. There had been some leakage around the drainage site for the first two or three weeks, but Nettie devised a rubber bandage device that solved the problem.

Unfortunately, intestinal dialysis wasn't working for Jimmy as efficiently as it seemed to have worked for those four patients of Dr. Clark and Associates, reported in the recent *Transactions of the ASAIO*. Jimmy's blood urea nitrogen was holding steady, but his blood creatinine values were gradually rising. Contrarily, his urine volumes were dropping. He was excreting only 200 to 300 ml of urine daily. These changes reflected further deterioration of his kidneys.

Over the next several months, more uremic symptoms emerged. His appetite dropped off. He was nauseated more frequently, and the itching returned. Shortly after beginning the intestinal dialysis, he had become more active, leaving home, from time to time, to visit some of his college buddies. But with the recurrence of uremic symptoms, he'd become more withdrawn, morose, obviously more depressed.

It had been only a week since I had seen him in my office, when I received a telephone call from Dr. Sherman, the surgeon who had constructed his intestinal loop.

"George, I saw your patient Jimmy wells in University last evening. He called my answering service right around midnight. He was having severe abdominal pain. Of course, I suspected the loop. It turned out his loop intussuscepted (telescoped on itself). I'm unsure why. He told me he'd been having some cramping, abdominal discomfort off and on for several days. Then, last night, it became severe and he called.

"Bottom line, I corrected the problem with a barium enema. Couldn't find any specific cause for the intussusception. Don't know if this has been a complication in other cases of isolated intestinal segments, but I'll do some research on this and let you know what I find."

"Thanks, Harry. I appreciate your help with Jimmy. He's a good kid who's gone through hell and back, a number of times."

"Yes, I know."

I called Jimmy the next day. He said he was doing okay. He'd had no further pain following the enema in the ER.

Because of his continued uremic symptoms, he had made the decision, on his own, to increase the length of time for dialyzing. He was planning to use the loop that night.

Less than a week later, I received a phone message from Nettie via my answering service. She wanted to let me know she was bringing Jimmy into the ER. He was having the same severe pain he'd had before. She had already called Dr. Sherman, who was to meet her there.

The loop had intussuscepted again. This time Dr. Sherman was able to relieve the intussusception manually. He called me afterwards and said, reluctantly, he felt that the loop would need to be reversed — reconnected to its original state. He was fearful that further intussusceptions could compromise Jimmy's intestinal circulation. The result could be gangrene or worse.

Jimmy was admitted to the hospital that night, and scheduled for surgery the next morning. The surgery was uncomplicated, and after a three-day stay he was discharged. Of course, his uremic symptoms would be returning. I was reluctant to discuss the need for restarting peritoneals. I was certain he would refuse to consider it.

A week later, I made a house call. I found Jimmy sitting in his La-Z-Boy chair watching a rerun of *Gunsmoke* on TV. He looked a bit pale. His face was puffy but his breathing was not labored and he was in good spirits. As soon as I walked in, he said, "Doc, no more peritoneals for me. So, don't even mention it. Let's just skip to the next subject. Best thing for us to do is just let me get back on the diet." He was composed and seemed committed to his decision about dialysis. He did admit that he stayed nauseated and didn't feel like eating.

"Doc, you and Nettie have given it a good try. Both of you've done everythin' you could to get me through this ... but, you know ... there comes a time when you just have to say enough's enough. And ... I think this is that time. No more dialysis treatments."

As Jimmy finished talking, Nettie walked in from the kitchen where she and her mother were cleaning up from dinner. She stood by Jimmy's chair. Tears rolled slowly down her cheeks, and her hands were shaking as she bent down and hugged Jimmy. She didn't say a word.

"But I tell you what I'm gonna do," Jimmy continued, his voice rising a bit. "I'm gonna get real strict on my diet. I promised Jake Davis, my old baseball coach—he dropped by yesterday—sorta' cheered me up a little, I guess. He made me promise him I wouldn't give up—said that wasn't me—to give up on anythin'. I told him that I was gonna hang in there as long as I could. I wasn't givin' up. So, that's when I decided to get serious about my diet and about my fluids."

Nettie stood up straight, stopped crying, and wiped the tears from her face. "Doc, Jake and about twenty of his and Jimmy's friends have started a fund for Jimmy. This Saturday, they're goin' house to house askin' for contributions ... hopin' to collect enough to help him prepare for his kidney transplant. I told them what he really needs is to be able to get treatments with an artificial kidney, to get him in good enough shape to be able to have the transplant surgery.

"And also, Doc," Nettie continued. "The local chapter of The International Brotherhood of Hospital Workers is gonna hold a benefit dance this same weekend at their Union Hall."

"That's great news, Nettie," I replied. "Let me know how the canvassing and the benefit dance go." I put my hand on Jimmy's shoulder and looked him in the eyes. "Jimmy, you sure you know what you'll need to do to get back on your diet. Do you want to talk to the dietitian again?"

"Nope, know it by heart, Doc," he quipped. "I'm just gonna have to have more determination to stick with it than I had before. I know I got lots'a people pullin' for me, and like I said ... I'm gonna give it everythin' I got."

I didn't mention dialysis to Jimmy. I certainly didn't want to bring up the possibility of hemodialysis, unless I had evidence that there was enough financial support to insure we could continue the procedure, once begun. Besides, I was reluctant to broach the subject of hemo dialyzing a patient with chronic renal disease with University.

I had not heard from the transplant team at Richmond, nor from any of the other programs I had contacted. The next few weeks would be critical for Jimmy. If he could stay on his diet and not become fluid overloaded, and if the benefit dance was successful in raising significant amounts of money, maybe arrangements could be made for using the artificial kidney at University Hospital. And maybe, just maybe, we would get the good news that a kidney transplant was eminent. A lot of maybes. But at least hope.

The dance and the door-to-door canvassing took place, as Nettie said. I never learned how successful they were.

Monday morning, two days after my house call, as I was starting rounds at University, my answering service called me. Nettie was on the phone. "Doc," she said. Her voice, faltering, and so low I could barely hear her. "Jimmy's passed." She was trying to get it out — what had happened — but the words just wouldn't come.

I said, "Nettie, don't try to tell me everything now. I'm so … so … sorry. It's been such a struggle for Jimmy, and for you and your mother. Such a struggle. Jimmy gave it all he could. We know that. It just seems it wasn't to be, that the odds were stacked against him. No matter what—"

Nettie broke in, her voice steadier now. "Doc, he jist didn't have the strength to keep on fightin'. He was jist wore out. He didn't want to let you down. He didn't want to let Doc Sherman down, me down, his friends down—didn't want to let any of us down. I knew he couldn't last much longer. Even though he talked brave when you an' him were together this past weekend." She wasn't crying now. She wanted to tell me everything.

"Doc, he went to bed last night around nine. But he was real restless. I could hear him tossin' and turnin' for a couple of hours, it seemed like. Then he went on to sleep. I checked on him three or four times before I went to bed, which was about twelve. Round seven this mornin', I went in his room. He wasn't breathin'. I knew he was gone. Poor little thing, he suffered so much. Now he can rest some. Now he can have some peace."

"Nettie, please let me know if there's anything I can do for you or your mother," I offered.

"Doc, you did all you could for Jimmy. You and Doctor Sherman both. Y'all gave it all, just like Jimmy did. Mom can't talk right now, but she wanted me to tell you how much she appreciated what you did for Jimmy. And Doc, don't you worry 'bout mom and me. We'll do alright. It'll take us awhile, but knowin' we did everything we could ... Well, that helps, at least some."

"You'll let me know when you'll have the service?" I said.

"Yes, we surely will."

JIMMY HAD BEEN in terminal renal failure for the last ten months, since early 1966. He died in January 1967. University Hospital received their artificial kidney, a Travenol U200A machine, a gift from the Women's Board, in November 1965.

Jimmy's funeral was held at the Mill Valley Baptist Church. Members of Jimmy's high school senior class, members of his college baseball team, Dr. Sherman, and I were honorary pallbearers.

I had difficulty agreeing with Nettie's assessment of my services. I was sad. I was depressed. I kept thinking about what could have been done differently.

CHAPTER 20

DIALYSIS AND TRANSPLANTATION

"(Arthur) Humphries was one of the first to preserve canine kidneys by combining constant perfusion with hypothermia" Organ **Donation and Transplantation after Cardiac Death. Editors: David Talbot and Anthony D'Alessandro, Oxford University Press; 2009, 37**

Over the last several years, I'd had a number of conversations with Dr. Arthur Humphries, an associate professor of surgery at MCG and a friend, about his ongoing work in successfully transplanting kidneys in dogs. I knew he was very interested in beginning a human kidney transplant program.

On several conversations, I had mentioned my patients with chronic renal failure. Several were end-stage and being peritoneally dialyzed on an as needed basis, as they awaited a kidney. He was aware of the difficulty I'd been having finding a transplant program willing to accept them. He intimated to me, it would not be long before he was ready to begin such a program himself.

In late 1967, I received a phone call from Dr. Jim Hudson, Chief of the Renal section at MCG. He asked if I would be interested in starting a hemodialysis program for patients with chronic renal failure at MCG's Talmadge Hospital. It would be a program that coordinated naturally with the expected forthcoming kidney transplant program.

I welcomed the opportunity. I would be able to keep my private medical practice and serve on the MCG faculty, as Assistant Clinical Professor in the Department of Medicine. More importantly, patients with chronic renal failure, finally, would have the assurance of reliable access to hemodialysis as a preparatory treatment procedure, before moving on to transplantation. At least, that was my vision. I told him I could start right away, if that suited him.

At the beginning of the year, Jeannie Carter, my office nurse, and I, along with technicians from MCG, set up the dialysis unit and began dialyzing patients at Talmadge. The solarium waiting room, on 5 West was transformed into a dialysis facility. We had one Travenol machine. Later, we acquired another machine from the Forest Hills VA Hospital in Augusta.

The State of Georgia assumed the financial responsibility for the dialysis treatments and later for the transplants. It wasn't until a decade or so later that the State allowed the federal government, along with private insurance companies, to participate in covering the costs of dialysis and transplantation.

We started with two patients, one on a Monday, Wednesday, Friday schedule, and the other on a Tuesday and Thursday schedule. We alternated the patients' schedule weekly. With the patients from MCG's renal service and with patients from my private practice, the dialysis unit filled up quickly.

In early spring of 1968, Larry Mitchell, from neighboring Langley, SC, was referred to me. Larry had far advanced chronic renal failure, secondary to glomerulonephritis. He was moderately uremic when I first saw him, and underwent two peritoneal dialyses before having an AV Teflon Silastic shunt created — in his arm — in preparation for hemodialysis.

He was started on a modified Giovannetti diet, blood pressure medications, multivitamins, and followed in the renal clinic at MCG. Larry was 26 years old and had a number of siblings who were considered to be potential donors. He was selected by Dr. Humphries to be the first MCG kidney transplant patient. His brother, Wayne, was chosen from six siblings as the most compatible donor.

In anticipation of his oncoming kidney transplant, Larry began regular hemodialysis in early summer of 1968. On August 28, same year, Larry received the kidney from his brother Wayne. The transplant was eminently successful. Larry's convalescence was uncomplicated, as was his brother's.

Larry was enjoying his newfound health and soon resumed working full time as a carpenter. He was doing many of the things, including water skiing, he had previously enjoyed prior to his illness.

In the fall of 1971, Larry and his wife began having marital problems. Relations between the two of them continued to worsen. In 1973, Larry was arrested for the murder of his wife. His defense argued that he was under the influence of multiple drugs that he was required to take to prevent his kidney from rejecting, and that he was not responsible for his actions. However, the jury convicted him and he was sentenced to life in the state prison in South Carolina. He died in the Columbia prison hospital in April 1976. I never knew whether or not the drugs Larry was taking played an integral part in his behavior.

CHAPTER 21

PRACTICING MEDICINE BY CONSENSUS

"They Decide Who Lives, Who Dies: Medical miracle puts moral burden on small committee" **Life magazine, 1962; 53 (November 9, 1962); 102-25 by Shana Alexander**

In the early 1960s, Belding Scribner and Associates in Seattle, pioneers in the field of dialysis, had strict criteria for determining which patients would receive the benefits of hemodialysis. A committee met regularly to go over candidates for dialytic treatment. I was vaguely aware of the composition of the committee, which had the daunting responsibility of determining who should live and who should die.

Later, I learned that there were actually two committees involved in the selection process. The first consisted of nephrologists who narrowed the selection process to exclude those patients with certain characteristics or conditions. For example: Persons over the age of forty-five were excluded. Children were not accepted, and diabetics were not even considered. Criteria changed over time.

The second committee, appointed by the Admission and Policies Commission of the Seattle Artificial Kidney Center, at Swedish Hospital consisted of six laymen and one physician — who was not a nephrologist—from the community. The makeup of this committee at its first meeting consisted of a spiritual leader, an attorney, a homemaker, a labor leader, a banker, a state government representative, and a surgeon. The first committee gave this committee lists of medically approved patients. The second committee, in turn, would have the final say as to who would be allowed to live, via this new source of life extension.

It was one thing to know about the groups of people who made decisions regarding who would live and who would die. It was a different experience entirely to be involved personally in making those decisions. Soon after the dialysis facility at the MCG was staffed and delivering dialysis treatments, I became part of a committee formed to evaluate patients for acceptance or rejection for dialysis. This committee consisted of staff from MCG and from the local community, somewhat similar to the makeup of the Seattle committees.

At our first meeting, I was discomfited by seeing and feeling how the selection process actually worked. First, there was an account of a patient's present illness. Then, questions were asked. What kind of work did he/she do? What education did this patient have? Was this patient emotionally stable enough to tolerate the demands of dialysis? How many dependents did the patient have? Did this patient have a value to the community greater than the other patients we discussed? What was the patient's income, religious affiliation, and criminal history?

Discussion ensued. After all questions were answered, we voted. The meeting was adjourned. There were more applicants than we could accept. The spots for dialysis were limited. Several "medically qualified" patients were not afforded the opportunity to extend their lives by hemodialysis. Now, I was a member of a life or death panel—disconcerting, at the very least.

Prior to working with the dialysis team at MCG, I had managed, one way or the other, to give every chronically uremic patient referred to me an opportunity to receive peritoneal dialysis. On occasions, they received only one dialysis. Some patients, usually those from outlying communities, decided not to return for follow up. Later, I would learn of their deaths from the newspapers, from their families, or from their referring doctor. A few patients had other medical complications that prevented them from returning for dialysis. Other patients were very compliant and continued following the dietary and limited dialysis treatments afforded them.

Fortunately, the referrals I received were not so many that I had to pick and choose amongst them. Now, with the opening of the dialysis facility at Talmadge Hospital, patients no longer were threatened by having to assume the financial burden of dialysis treatments. The State of Georgia assumed that responsibility. I anticipated that my private patients, along with others already followed by other faculty physicians at MCG, would have ready access to dialytic treatment.

Quickly, it became apparent that not all patients needing dialysis would have that opportunity. The pool of patients with end-stage renal disease had expanded. There was a finite number of spots for hemodialysis patients. Some method of admittance to the center was required — hence the selection committee and the practice of medicine by consensus. Of necessity, some patients — to put it realistically — would be left to die. Although I had considerable misgivings about our method of patient selection, I accepted it as a necessary evil.

THE MCG TRANSPLANT PROGRAM that started with Wayne Mitchell donating one of his kidneys to his brother, Larry, was up and running. Over the next year, Dr. Humphries successfully transplanted three more patients. The dialysis unit added a second shift. More patients had access to dialysis. Still, some patients died because of the limited availability of dialysis and transplant options.

Over the months following Larry Mitchell's transplant, the dialysis facility at MCG, continued to serve as a holding unit for patients awaiting transplantation. We continued using the same selection formula. I was becoming increasingly disillusioned and saddened by our selection process.

Using diet and intermittent peritoneal dialysis, I continued to manage the patients I had been following in my private practice, who were not candidates for transplantation. Robert Jackson had no potential donors and would not be considered for dialysis/transplantation before other patients with related — potential — donors. Still, he was being managed by these measures, and doing well enough — all things considered.

Lorine Thompson, another patient from my private practice, was fortunate enough to be accepted on the MCG dialysis program. Lorine was in her early thirties. Her obstetrician referred her to me when he found albumin in her urine, and a high BUN.

Subsequently, her workup revealed creatinine clearances in the range of 10 to 12 ml/min. Her kidneys were bilaterally small. She was hypertensive and retaining excess fluid. Her spun urine sediment showed elements consistent with chronic glomerular nephritis.

For the last five to six months, she had been on a modified Giovannetti diet along with salt and potassium restriction, and had reached a point where dialysis was indicated. She underwent several peritoneals at University Hospital before I asked Dr. Humphries to evaluate her for a kidney transplant.

Mrs. Thompson had ten siblings and Dr. Humphries felt she would be a good candidate for transplantation. As it turned out, only one of her siblings, her younger sister, Wanda, was a match.

Mrs. Thompson was a good patient. Her temperament was much like that of Mrs. Kimble. She was always cooperative, appreciative, and never complained of any of the inconveniences she bore during dialysis or her workup for the transplant.

She easily fulfilled the panel's criteria for dialysis/transplantation. She was dialyzed on a regular basis at MCG, until she received her sister's kidney in September 1969.

Mrs. Thompson's kidney transplant was the sixth in MCG's program. Like the other five transplants, hers was successful. She had regained her vigor and strength, and was thoroughly enjoying her newly recovered health. Then, on January 25, 1970, tragedy struck again. Lorine suffered a catastrophic stroke, unrelated to the transplant surgery. She died three days later. The family was devastated. Her other caregivers and I were saddened in disbelief.

CHAPTER 22

CHRONIC HEMODIALYSIS

"The concept of applying HD (Hemodialysis) to patients with end-stage-renal-failure (ESRF), first pioneered by Alwal in Sweden as far back as 1948, became a reality in 1960 when Scribner, Quniton, et al. designed an external arteriovenous by pass ... which allowed a permanent access to the bloodstream ..." **Renal replacement therapy by hemodialysis: an overview. Nephrol Ther.2009 Jul: 5 (4) Jacobs C.**

Two older patients I was following, Howard Dubinion and Julia Kanovich, because of their ages, were not candidates for transplantation. Unfortunately, this meant they would not be considered for hemodialysis, not as long as more suitable transplant patients were still on the waiting list.

The Scribner shunt was still considered the definitive vascular access for chronic hemodialysis. But a newer method for gaining access to the circulation, the Cimino-Brescia Arteriovenous fistula, would soon over take the Scribner shunt as the favored access. Hemodialysis for chronic progressive renal failure was entering mainstream medicine.

WAYNE WILLIS, a forty-six year old mechanical engineer who worked at McDougall Industries, just outside

Waynesboro, was one of the new patients with chronic renal disease, recently referred to me. Wayne had been a patient of Dr. Wiley Gilcrist, his local physician, for the last fifteen or so years. He was diagnosed with chronic renal disease about a year ago, when his BUN and serum creatinine began rising. He'd had longstanding hypertension and was on several antihypertensive drugs when I first examined him.

Even though his creatinine clearances were low, he had only a few symptoms of uremia. His Hgb was 10 gm%, he complained of fatigue over the last few months, and he had begun to itch.

I started him on a limited protein Giovannetti type diet, restricted his sodium and potassium, and saw him at regular intervals in my office. Within the last two months, his clearances had dropped significantly. He was nearing end-stage. I admitted him to University three times during this period because of his loss of appetite and persistent nausea. I dialyzed him on two of those occasions.

During his last hospitalization, while receiving peritoneal dialysis, he asked a lot of questions about the Travenol dialysis machine stored in the same room, next to his bed. I explained the theory of dialysis to him, and pointed out the main features of the machine: the blood lines connected to the dialysis coil, the arterial line taking blood from the patient, running it through the coil immersed in the dialysate in the tub, filtering out the impurities, and returning the cleansed blood back to the patient.

"Doctor," he said. "The machine seems very straightforward. I mean, from a purely mechanical standpoint. Do you know how much one of those costs?"

I said, "Somewhat less than $2000."

"You know, Doctor, I believe I could build one myself for a whole lot less."

"It's interesting you say this, Mr. Willis. I've thought the same thing for the last couple of years."

Mr. Willis had excellent hospitalization insurance through his company. But he was not a candidate for transplantation because of his age and lack of related donors. I never brought up his case for consideration in our discussions at MCG.

It was during this period that I began considering how patients like Wayne Willis or Julia Kanovich, or Howard Dubinion might receive hemodialysis. I thought this could be done, as I had tried to do with peritoneal dialysis, in a location other than a hospital. Perhaps, I thought, in an office with a room for a dialysis machine.

I envisioned patients being trained in an outpatient facility to dialyze at home, awaiting the definitive treatment for chronic renal failure; still, to my mind, a kidney transplant. If the criteria for transplantation changed, and if transplantation facilities became more readily assessable, these patients, and others like them, could be shifted easily into transplant programs.

With my attending the dialysis facility at MCG in the morning for several hours, then making rounds at three hospitals, and trying to be in my office for morning patients by eleven o'clock I was being stretched thin. Additionally, I had become involved with a group of physicians exploring the possibility of building a new, physician-owned and operated, hospital. All this left me little time for a personal life.

I felt I could care for more patients, especially older ones not eligible for transplantation, if I had more autonomy. The MCG dialysis center was running very smoothly now and was at capacity. The nursing personnel and other staff members had developed a well-managed and efficient treatment center. I had no question in my mind that the facility would continue functioning this way if I left.

I was still having difficulty accepting our method of patient selection for admission to the center although I was fully aware that this was as good a method of selection as conditions allowed in the late 1960s.

I spoke with Jim Hudson about my idea of setting up an out-of-hospital dialysis center for patients who were non-candidates for transplantation, a setting for patients with chronic renal failure who would be trained for home dialysis.

At the time, he told me he thought outpatient dialysis clinics would play a major role in the management of chronic renal disease in the future, that most such patients would be coming to these clinics for dialysis treatments on a regular basis.

"Jim, you really think patients would take six to eight hours a day, three days a week, out of their lives, and come to a clinic to be hooked up to a dialysis machine?" I asked incredulously.

"Yep, that's what will happen, I believe."

I expected home dialysis to be the wave of the future. There, patients could bide their time, dialyzing on their own schedule, waiting to be called by a kidney transplant program. Earlier, Dr. Scribner's Seattle clinic and the Spokane Kidney Center had adopted a policy that all patients with chronic renal failure reaching end-stage disease would be either home dialyzed or transplanted.

By the early 1970s, some 90% of dialysis patients at Scribner's Seattle clinic were dialyzing at home. These demographics were to change dramatically over the ensuing decades. The renal transplant programs were unable to meet the demands of the increasing numbers of patients with chronic renal failure who presented themselves to both transplant physicians and nephrologists, especially after the implementation of the Renal Medicare Program. Outpatient dialysis centers became the "preferred" treatment modality for a majority of patients with end stage renal disease. Dr. Hudson was prescient.

CHAPTER 23

THE MOVE

"In 1963, one of the abstracts we submitted for the Ninth ASAIO Congress entitled 'Hemodialysis at Home: Utilizing Domestic Electric Washing Machine' by Y. Nose and J. Mikami was rejected." **Home hemodialysis: a crazy idea in 1963: a memoir, Nose, Y. ASAIO J. 2000 Jan-Feb; 46(1): 13**

The office John Phinizy and I had redesigned on Central Ave was working well for his and most of my patients, but not for my patients who needed dialysis. I needed an office in which I could set up an artificial kidney — hemodialysis — machine and offer dialysis to those patients.

I resigned my position as director of the MCG dialysis facility later in the year, and in February 1969, I vacated the office that John Phinizy and I designed, built, and shared for the last four years. I moved to 1445 Harper Street, within walking distance to both Talmadge and University Hospitals.

The new office had a small room, actually a utility closet, which I planned to use for dialysis. Although small, it had water, a sink, and electricity. It was just large enough for a dialysis machine and a nurse.

It was sad for me to separate from John. He was a good friend, close associate, and had been so generous in helping me start my practice. Our relationship lasted long after he moved from Augusta to practice solo, in Barnwell, South Carolina. He, in good humor, told people who asked why I moved, that I divorced him for a dialysis machine. This was more or less accurate, I suppose.

I remained closely associated with MCG, making rounds with medical students, meeting with the renal and surgery groups to discuss dialysis, transplantation patients, and issues, while continuing as a preceptor to medical students.

I set about equipping my office on Harper Street for hemodialysis. I wanted a machine similar to the Travenol model we used at MCG. But I couldn't afford to spend the several thousand dollars necessary to purchase the Travenol machine.

The Seattle group started their dialysis program using the Kiil dialyzer, and although the Kiil did not require a blood pump, it was, in my opinion, more cumbersome and more complicated to use than the Travenol to which I had become accustomed.

Beginning in the 1940s, Dr. Willem Johan Kolff, often referred to as the "father of modern dialysis," because of his seminal work in the field of dialysis, had used Maytag washing machines for dialysis in the mid 1960s. He used them until lawyers from the Maytag Company, worrying over lawsuits, forbid him to continue.

Dr. Kolff always contended that dialysis should be as simple to perform and as economical as possible. I felt the same way. In reviewing the literature on hemodialysis for that era, I found it interesting that several other physicians, working in the same field, also began dialyzing by modifying washing machines. Frugality was the watchword during that period.

I already owned a Maytag washer. My wife, Gail, and I purchased it in 1960 when I was a medical resident at MCG. We weren't using it now. We had a newer, more efficient model. However, being a pack rat, I never discarded that Maytag. I had stored it in a closet at home.

Now, I reclaimed it from storage, brought it to Harper Street, and began transforming it from a machine that washed clothes to one that cleansed blood. I removed the wringer and the agitator and carefully determined the volume of water the tank would hold. I scratched a line on the inside of the tank marking the level for 100 liters, the same volume as in the Travenol tank.

I secured a canister, for holding dialysis coils, and attached it to the inside of the washer with an improvised sling. I bought an aquarium pump to which I attached tubing. The tubing, in turn, was attached to the coil, at the bottom of the canister and through which the dialysate would flow. The

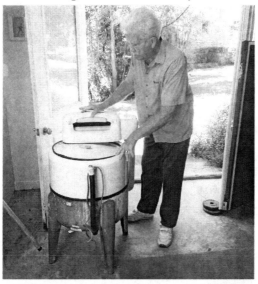

Dr. Van Giesen with a Maytag like the one used in his office

pump delivered approximately 500 ml/min, the same as the Travenol machine's dialysis flow rate.

The costs for having a machine that performed the functions of a commercial dialysis machine were minimal. The aquarium pump cost $10. Another $2 or $3 for the tubing and metal attachment for the canister. I purchased a used SigmaMotor finger pump, for moving the blood through the dialysis circuit, for $12. And I bought an adjustable, standing, reading lamp to beam over the side of the tank, to keep the dialysate warm. The coils, dialysis tubing, and dialysate concentrate were the most expensive items of the entire setup.

I had decided that Wayne Willis, should be the first patient offered a spot in the Augusta Dialysis Center on Harper Street. Mr. Willis' clearances had dropped gradually over the last six months, and now, were in the same range as those of Mrs. Kimble, during the last days of her life. This concerned me. Mr. Willis had tolerated, without any complaints or protestations, the drastic changes in his way of life: the rigid dietary and fluid restrictions, the multiple drugs he was taking to control his blood pressure, and his lack of energy.

His Hgb had dropped to 8 gm%. On two occasions recently, peritoneal dialysis relieved the worst of his uremic symptoms, but he needed longer reprieves, requiring more efficient and frequent dialytic treatments. During his last hospitalization, I explained to him and his wife, Donna, the issues he was facing.

"Mr. Willis," I said, trying to sound as matter-of-factly as I could. "I feel it's time to consider changing your present regimen."

Mr. Willis was a very stoic person. In spite of his illness, he continued to work every day except Sundays. He had been trained as a mechanical engineer, finally receiving his BS degree at Augusta Tech, after years of night schooling. He entered the real work force world when he was in his mid thirties. McDougall Industries had come to depend on him.

"Doctor," he said. "You mean we should change the medications I'm taking?"

"No, not the meds. For the time being, we'll just leave them as they are. But, you remember last year, when I told you about the opening of the dialysis facility at Talmadge?"

"Yes, I recall you talking about that."

"Well, I mentioned patients would be accepted if they were potential candidates for transplant; but, because of your age, you would not be a candidate, at least not at that time. I also explained that, even if you were considerably younger, you still might not be a candidate for transplant because of your potential donor's age. You said your brother was in his fifties, I believe."

"I do remember you telling me this."

"I realize that you're not having much difficulty sticking with your present regimen, but your kidney clearances are very low. They have reached a level where I am concerned that things could go wrong suddenly.

"This diet you're on works as long as you have a modicum of kidney function left. Below that, in some patients, bad things can happen. Blood levels of potassium can rise quickly, and can cause heart disturbances and other serious problems. I don't want to scare you. You've done really well about staying on your diet and controlling your liquid intake. But, I don't want you to have any of the untoward consequences of this diet. You should be on a regular dialysis program, but not peritoneal dialysis. You should be on hemodialysis — using an artificial kidney."

"But," he hesitated momentarily, "you said, since I wouldn't be able to get a transplant, I wouldn't be accepted at Talmadge for dialysis?"

"Mr. Willis," I continued, "that's correct. However, I have a machine, right now, in my office, that replicates the functions of the artificial kidney. It's like the one at University and the one we're using at Talmadge. I'd like you to come over to the office and take a look at it when you leave the hospital tomorrow. We could begin using it right away."

The next day, after he was discharged from University, Mr. Willis and his wife stopped by my office. I had finished morning rounds and was reading yesterday's mail. Aside from looking a little pale, Mr. Willis showed few signs of chronic kidney failure.

I led them into the back utility closet, converted into a dialysis room, to view the machine. "As you can see," I said, "this is a very basic artificial kidney. Well, to be honest, it's a Maytag washer with the agitator and wringer removed, and modified to function as a dialysis machine. It works like this: the tank is filled with tap water adjusted to body temperature. A concentrate of glucose and minerals is added to the water.

A commercial coil made of cellophane is set in a canister, which is placed in the solution. The tank holds the solution, which now is the dialysate.

"I don't want you to think that using a washing machine for dialysis is just some cockamamie idea of mine. It's not. It's not an original idea of mine, either." I told them about Dr. Kolff's reputation as one of the pioneers of modern dialysis, and his original work with artificial kidneys in the 1940s, continuing through the '50s, and into the early '60's. At the Cleveland clinic, he successively trained several dozen patients for home dialysis, using modified Maytag washers.

Mr. Willis quickly chimed in. "Seems like a good idea to me, Doctor. Now what about the vascular access you mentioned the other day in the hospital?" He was studying the makeshift dialysis machine intensely, as though visualizing himself connected to it.

"Well, you would need a shunt, which is made of Teflon and Silastic components, and surgically implanted in your arm. One section would be threaded into an artery and the other into a vein, creating an arterial venous, AV, fistula. This would allow you to be connected to the dialysis machine as needed. When you were not being dialyzed the arterial and venous sections are reconnected. Your arm is then bandaged and you go about your business as usual. Of course, it will be very important that you keep the shunt clean, so it doesn't get infected, and be careful to keep from injuring that arm."

Mrs. Willis had been standing quietly at her husband's side, listening carefully to what I was telling them. She seemed stunned. She was looking straight ahead, her eyes wide open like a deer caught in the headlights. "Doctor Van," she spoke very softly, not looking directly at me. "I ... I just don't understand. All this is happening so fast. How long would Wayne have to do this?"

"For six hours," I said. "And ... I'd suggest twice a week, at the start."

"But how long will he need to do this? I mean weeks, months, or what? And ... you think he needs to start right away? Isn't this a risky procedure?"

"Mrs. Willis," I said, reassuringly. "The risk for him is to not start dialysis. His kidneys are functioning at a very low level, a potentially dangerous level. His condition could worsen abruptly. As for how long he'll need to stay on dialysis, unfortunately, it'll be as long as it takes until he can receive a kidney transplant."

Mrs. Willis said she was feeling a little weak. She sat down, closed her eyes, and rested her head in her hands. Mr. Willis was walking around the machine, checking out all aspects of its assembly, seemingly taking mental notes of how this hybrid machine was put together. He walked over to where his wife was sitting and rested his hand lightly on her shoulder. He whispered, "Not to worry, Donna. I trust Dr. Van Giesen. He says it's important that I start on dialysis right away. I'm ready to do it. Things have a way of working out." She looked up and nodded her head. A tiny smile on her lips faded quickly.

I asked Dr. Sherman if he would evaluate Mr. Willis for a shunt. He was able to schedule the surgery later in the week. He found Mr. Willis to have easily assessable vessels, and as Mr. Willis was right handed, he placed the shunt in his left forearm.

I had made prior arrangements of engaging an LPN from University Hospital to work for me the two days that Mr. Willis would be needing dialysis. Essie Farrington was on permanent night shift on Barrett 2, and was one of the nurses I depended on for acute hospital dialysis procedures.

She said it would be easy for her to come to my office after the night shift, and dialyze Mr. Willis for the six hours he required, that she never tried to go to sleep until much later in the day.

I arranged for Mr. Willis to begin dialysis on a Monday and Thursday schedule. He wanted to come as early as possible. That was fine with me. I'd be able to get the dialysis going before I started morning rounds. My plan was to train both him and his wife to dialyze at home.

One week after the Scribner shunt had been placed in his forearm, Mr. Willis arrived promptly at eight o'clock for his first dialysis. Essie Farrington and I, repeatedly, had gone over the protocol for dialyzing on the Maytag.

THERE BEING NO MECHANISM in the Maytag dialysis machine for heating the dialysate, ordinary tap water was brought to body temperature by mixing hot and cold water from the faucets. In those days, no one gave much consideration to treating the water. The Savannah River, from which Augusta obtained its water supply, was found to be very low in mineral content. This was considered ideal for dialysis.

The temperature was kept constant by adjusting the distance of the lamp from the dialysate. The thermometer hung in the dialysate throughout the treatment. The temperature was checked and charted every 15 minutes throughout the procedure. A manometer, taken from a blood pressure cuff, monitored pressure in the venous lines.

The patient was weighed at the beginning and end of dialysis. At the beginning of the dialysis, it was very important to insure that the dialysis concentrate had been added to the water — now dialysate or bath — in the tank. This was checked by adding a drop of blood to a test tube of dialysate. If the dialysate in the test tube became cloudy, that would indicate that the concentrate had been added. If the dialysate showed no cloudiness, the red blood cells were being broken down (hemolyzed); that was evidence that the concentrate had not been added and the dialysis could not begin. The test tube was taped to the side of the machine. Dialysis was never started until this test had been done and recorded.

There were other safety measures. The dialysis nurse kept two surgical clamps attached to her gown, ready to clamp lines should one come apart, or some other catastrophe occur — such as a coil rupturing. The main concern was being able to terminate the dialysis and prevent blood loss from the patient by clamping the arterial line and returning as much blood back to the patient via the venous line as possible. The nurse was in the room with the patient at all times during the dialysis procedure.

The dialysate was drained and reconstituted at the end of two hours, and again after four hours. The tank was emptied completely by turning on the drain pump of the washer at the end of the dialysis, and sterilized with Clorox. Prior to each new dialysis, it was tested for traces of Clorox.

MR. WILLIS SEATED himself in the La-Z-Boy recliner next to the Maytag. I removed the dressing from his arm. The shunt had a loud bruit, indicating it was functioning as designed. An IV of glucose and saline was started to fill the lines and the coil. The tubing was fed into the SigmaMotor pump. The arterial and venous lines were connected to the arterial and venous tubing attached to the coil. Heparin was injected through the tubing to keep the blood from clotting. The pump was turned on, and dialysis began.

Mr. Willis' blood pressure was monitored every minute for the first fifteen minutes, then every thirty minutes thereafter. The speed of the SigmaMotor pump was gradually increased. There was no suction effect in the arterial line, indicating an adequate arterial flow of blood.

Mr. Willis did not appear to be anxious as we started the dialysis. He asked if he could read a *Popular Science* magazine laying on a small table next to his chair. After about fifteen to twenty minutes, the magazine fell from his lap. His eyes were closed. He was asleep.

We ran the dialysis for only two hours the first treatment, four hours the next time, and the full six hours from then on. We were extremely careful about increasing the blood flow — turning up the SigmaMotor pump — during dialysis. Changes in the rate were made in small increments.

For the most part, we had no untoward problems with Mr. Willis' dialyses. After six weeks of twice-weekly treatments, we changed to a Monday, Wednesday, and Friday schedule. This frequency was becoming the new standard.

Mr. Willis' insurance covered his dialysis treatments as long as they were reported as office visits. In those days, I had just raised my office visit fees from $7.50 to $10. I didn't charge extra for the dialysis. His, and many insurance companies, had not accepted hemodialysis — much less hemodialysis in an out of hospital facility — as anything less than an experimental procedure. Expenses above those covered by his insurance were paid from the special kidney account I'd set up a number of years ago.

Mr. Willis continued to dialyze at the Harper Street Clinic, which now was Augusta Dialysis Center, without incident. When he began a thrice-weekly schedule, Essie Farrington gave me a two-week notice that she would not be able to work the longer hours this change required.

I tried to "steal" other nurses from the local hospitals, but was unable to induce any to leave their more secure jobs. My wife, Gail, saved the day. A registered nurse by training, she had been away from nursing for several years. But she insisted on helping out in the clinic with Mr. Willis, until I could find other help. She hoped soon.

MR. WILLIS HAD BEEN dialyzing for about three months. Most of the time he had no problems during dialysis. On occasions he had cramps, but these were usually quickly relieved when he licked salt from the back of his hand. When he had too much fluid, a screw clamp on the venous line was tightened, and extra fluid was removed slowly during the dialysis.

His blood pressures were running in safe ranges and he had adapted well to living with dialysis. His company allowed him a leave of absence for six weeks while he was adjusting to his different lifestyle. After that, his work schedule was changed so he could have mornings off, Mondays, Wednesday, and Fridays. He made up hours lost by working longer on non-dialysis days. His only complaint was not having the stamina he used to have. His Hgb hovered around 7 to 7.5 gm%.

In the early years, essentially all dialysis patients were anemic. When their Hgb dropped too low they received blood transfusions. Some patients saw their Hgb levels rise with testosterone administration. But most patients learned to live with less than normal Hgb levels.

ERYTHROPOIETIN (EPO), the hormone that stimulates red cell production, is primarily secreted by the kidneys. In chronic renal failure there is not enough circulating EPO to stimulate the bone marrow to produce red blood cells. EPO eventually was synthesized, but wasn't available for administration to dialysis patients until the late 1980s.

Some patients tolerated low Hgb levels better than others. I had one patient who refused blood transfusions. His Hgb levels stayed in the 7 gm% range, yet he had adapted so well to his anemia that he was able to swim long distances regularly — in both the ocean and in his gym pool.

ONE MORNING after his dialysis, Mr. Willis stopped me as I was leaving the dialysis room. "Doctor, I've been working on a little project I'd like to show you. I've got it in the back of my pickup."

"Yes, I'd like to see it," I replied, wondering what his project was.

We walked to the back lot where he had parked his '62 Chevy truck. In the bed was a large tub with various attachments, both electrical and mechanical. It resembled my Maytag dialysis machine. I was surprised — and impressed. He had built his own dialysis machine!

"Doctor, I've been working on this in the plant shop," he said. "After I got a good understanding of the workings of a dialysis machine, and after I'd had some runs on yours, I figured I could improve on both yours and Travenol's design. No offense intended, you understand." He was pleasant but strictly business, as usual.

"No, Mr. Willis, no offense," I replied, smiling. "I need all the engineering advice I can get when it comes to designing and constructing a dialysis machine."

He continued, "Since my insurance company informed me they wouldn't cover the cost of an artificial kidney, I figured I'd build my own. I also figured if I had a dialysis machine at home, and could get Donna used to seeing it, the quicker I could start dialyzing there. You know, Donna's pretty scared of this whole business: the machine, the blood, the shunt, everything associated with it."

"Yes, I know. It seems she postpones her training every week."

"I've had my machine sitting in our bedroom for the last couple of weeks, and Donna seems to be adjusting to the idea of me eventually dialyzing at home. What I'd like to do, is leave the machine here with you for a while. And let's give it a few trial runs, see if you think it would be safe to use at home."

"Sounds like a good idea. Let's see about taking it off your truck. Can the two of us manage it?"

My afternoon patients were filling my office and I was already a half-hour late in seeing my appointments. Quickly, we unloaded his machine. It was lighter than the Maytag. We rolled it through the back door and into a corner of the break room. The little dialysis room wasn't large enough to accommodate another artificial kidney.

I told Mr. Willis I would take good care of his prototype artificial kidney. I suggested he come in early next dialysis day and we'd give it a tryout.

Mr. Willis' dialysis machine was, in fact, an improvement over mine. For example, he had added a thermostatically controlled heating element, and instead of a finger pump for circulating the blood, he fashioned his own roller pump. Also, it had wheels. In one way, it was even better than the Travenol model we were using at Talmadge and University. It was smaller and took up less space, better for home use.

When Mr. Willis came for his next dialysis, the Willis machine was sitting in the spot previously occupied by my Maytag. We started his dialysis on the "Willis." It worked as designed. His six-hour dialysis was uneventful. Gail told me the machine was easier to use than the Maytag. At the least, she didn't have to worry as much about maintaining the proper temperature.

Over the next several months, Mr. Willis continued dialyzing on his machine. His shunt was holding out. He was keeping meticulous care of it. There was never any sign of infection.

It took Mrs. Willis about another month before she showed up for her training. By this time, Mr. Willis was thoroughly acquainted with the details and possible complications of dialysis in general, and of his machine in particular. He told me, on several occasions, that he was sure he could manage the dialysis by himself if he had to. That he only needed someone to help him start and finish the treatment.

He said he wanted to spare Donna the ordeal of "having to put up with my incapacity." Donna, however, was a quick learner and soon became proficient as a dialysis nurse/technician. She learned when to flatten out the recliner and when to adjust the rate of the intravenous solution to maintain blood pressures at optimum levels. She overcame her dread of dialysis and after about three months of running the sessions, with Gail's supervision, she told us she felt she was ready to dialyze at home. We agreed with her.

Donna's training lasted a little over three months. We never pushed to get Mr. Willis out of the office and into a home setting. By then, I was confident that he and Donna would be able to successfully manage home dialysis. Gail and I went home with them on several occasions to help them decide on the best place for him to dialyze.

Mr. Willis had a small room that he used as his study. He felt this would suit him best, but it had no water source or drain. However, it was adjacent to a half bath in the hall. He said that running a hose to the machine and another from the drain into the sink would solve that problem. The three of us agreed that this arrangement should work. Later, Mr. Willis had the water source and drain brought into the room.

For their first dialysis away from the security of my office, Gail and I again went home with them. Donna, very capably, made all the right connections, started the IV drip appropriately, and monitored the dialysis in a professional manner. I stayed for the first hour, during which time Mr. Willis' vital signs remained stable. Gail stayed for the entire dialysis. They had no problems the remainder of the treatment.

I arranged for Mr. Willis to buy his dialysis coils and other supplies from me at cost. After several months of home dialysis, the Willises invited their insurance representative to visit them while Mr. Willis was being dialyzed. The agent, observing the dialysis treatment, was impressed. He spent the next several weeks trying to convince his home office that a broad interpretation of the major medical clause should allow the Willises to be reimbursed for the costs of the dialysis equipment.

In a few weeks, I received a phone call from the insurer. They wanted to know how long I expected to keep Mr. Willis on dialysis. I gave them the same answer I'd given Mrs. Willis. Until a kidney transplant program accepted him. No doubt, the insurance company wasn't pleased with my answer. But likely, they felt that the positive public relations outweighed the negative financials of covering Mr. Willis' dialysis supplies. His insurance remained intact as long as he continued on dialysis.

Now, the Willises would be able to maintain a semblance of normal life while awaiting transplantation centers to modify their criteria for transplanting kidneys into older patients. I had already begun making enquiries around the country for him.

CHAPTER 24

SELF CARE

"The most important advice I can give a patient is to get involved: get involved in your own healthcare, get involved and stay involved."

Mandy Trolinger, MS, RD, former dialysis patient, two time transplant patient, and dialysis dietitian D&T; 2007 In Their Words PATIENT PARTICIPATION IN THE DIALYSIS SETTING in Dialysis and Transplantation 2008

Robert Jackson, Julia Kanovich, and Howard Dubinion were not thriving on their dietary and intermittent peritoneal dialysis regimens, but they remained relatively free of the more intolerable symptoms of a full uremic state. Robert, because of his higher blood pressures, lower renal clearances, and his inability to maintain a dry weight, was more vulnerable to the complications of terminal renal failure than the other two.

Robert's kidneys, having shown some improvement following his early dialyses, were deteriorating again. His urine output was diminishing and diuretics were ineffective. He'd had no further seizures and his eye grounds showed no evidence of the hemorrhages, exudates, and papilledema he had at the beginning of his treatments. I had searched for anything that might aid Robert in maintaining a dry weight —

anything that might allow him a better chance of lowering his blood pressure.

MCG's Talmadge Hospital, had a sauna on the sixth floor in the metabolic ward. Dr. Al Carr, in charge of the metabolic unit, allowed me to use the sauna for Robert on an as needed basis. I arranged for him to begin thirty-minute sauna treatments once a week. Later, I increased his treatments to three times a week. Robert lived nearby and was able to continue these sessions regularly.

The sauna treatments did remove some fluid and improve his mood, but his blood pressure remained too high. Robert was receiving peritoneal dialyses about every three weeks. He tolerated the intermittent puncture technique at this frequency. Baxter/Travenol continued to supply peritoneal supplies, including disposable trays and dialysis solutions, and University continued to provide the room on Barrett 2 for dialysis.

I soon learned that the insurance policy of Robert's grandmother didn't cover any of his dialysis treatments. Even though he needed more frequent dialyses, I felt that was not an option under the circumstances.

I wanted to start him on hemodialysis as soon as I could. Gail needed to be back at home with our two children—Diane, eleven and Eddie, nine—but she agreed to stay and help Robert start on dialysis.

In the meantime, I'd hired Edith Harrison, an LPN from St. Joseph Hospital. Edith had been on rotating shifts and was looking for a strictly daytime position. She wasn't skilled in hemodialysis, but she had helped with several of my patients undergoing peritoneal dialyses at St. Joseph. She was a very competent nurse and dedicated to her profession. I was confident that she would learn the technique of hemodialysis without difficulty.

During the time Mr. and Mrs. Willis were being trained for home dialysis, I had several talks with Robert Jackson about starting him on hemodialysis soon. I knew that he would not be able to dialyze at home. His grandmother suffered a stroke a number of years ago, and was physically unable to manage the dialysis machine. From the beginning, I knew that Robert would remain an outpatient on dialysis, until he could be transferred to a center willing and able to give him a cadaver transplant.

Although Brescia and Cimino's AV fistula technique of connecting an artery to a vein had been used successfully in patients with chronic renal failure for the last several years, I was hesitant to use it until I was satisfied of its superiority over the Scribner shunt. I asked Dr. Sherman to see Robert for shunt evaluation. He was able to set him up for the surgery within a matter of days. Robert started dialysis treatments a week later.

Robert's shunt did not function as well as that of Wayne Willis. It clotted and had to be cleared on a number of occasions. Nonetheless, I continued to work with it for the next five to six months. Eventually, because of these complications, the shunt was removed and an AV fistula was created in its place.

Robert's dialysis went much smoother following the creation of his AV fistula. He had been dialyzing via the fistula for about three months when one morning, as I was leaving the dialysis room to make hospital rounds, he stopped me. "Doctor VG, how 'bout me learning to stick myself? Ms. Harrison does a good job—I really don't feel the stick anymore—but, I'd like to try it myself."

"I don't have a problem with that," I replied. "How about you, Ms. Harrison?"

"I'm all for it," she replied.

Over the next several weeks, Robert learned the technique of cannulating his veins and soon became proficient in doing so. He was dialyzing now for six hours on Monday, Wednesday, and Friday.

As he began taking more and more of an interest in his dialysis, his physical and mental condition improved, as did his blood chemistries. His dialysis schedule allowed him the freedom that the GG diet and intermittent peritoneals didn't.

Robert wanted a job. He felt good enough to work, but because he was on dialysis, nobody wanted to hire him. He was coming to dialysis about thirty minutes prior to starting the procedure. He started setting up his machine under the supervision of Ms. Harrison. Soon, except for coming on and off, he was managing the entire dialysis on his own. He, like Mr. Willis, had become a self-care dialysis patient.

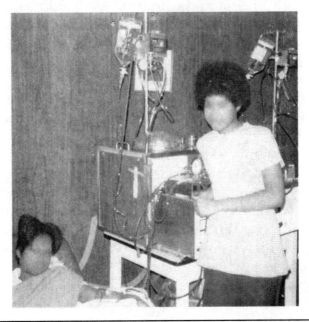

Patient and family member in dialysis center on 15th street. Faces blurred to protect their privacy.

JULIA KANOVICH, along with Howard Dubinion, remained on the GG diet and intermittent peritoneal dialysis regimen. Both were relatively free of uremic symptoms, but Mr. Dubinion's clearances were dropping into the danger zone, and I wanted to start him on hemodialysis as soon as it was feasible.

Only Tuesdays and Thursdays were available for dialyzing. Saturdays were open, but at the time, I didn't feel that our dialyzing patients six days a week was an option. I wasn't ready to commit myself to the obligation of working every weekend. I was working over eighty hours a week as it was. The bottom line: After arranging for a Scribner shunt, I started Mr. Dubinion on a twice weekly routine, running the dialyses six and a half hours each treatment session.

Mr. Dubinion's shunt did not function satisfactorily from the beginning. Clotting was the main problem. After repeated declottings, we managed to keep it open by starting low dose Coumadin—a drug to prevent intravascular clotting.

Now, the Augusta Dialysis Center's Harper Street clinic was full. I knew Robert Jackson would not be going home on dialysis, at least until someone other than his grandmother could be trained to aid in the treatments. I had it in mind that Mr. Dubinion could and would be home trained. Little did I realize the enormity of that endeavor.

Ellen Dubinion was one year younger than her husband. A gray haired, slightly overweight, grandmother of five, she seemed very distracted, or maybe even fearful, whenever she accompanied her husband for office appointments. She was a very quiet lady. Very reserved. She had been quite taken aback when I explained to them the seriousness of Howard's kidney condition during one of their earlier visits.

"Not Howard, not Howard," she exclaimed repeatedly. Then burst into tears. "He's such a good man, such a good person. He doesn't deserve this."

Mrs. Dubinion worked as a seamstress in Segar's Industries, a garment factory on Highway 51, a short distance from Augusta. She had altered her work hours so she could drive him to and from dialysis on Tuesdays and Thursdays. But she made it a point to leave the office as soon as she dropped Howard off. She would drive to her sister's home, in west Augusta, and stay there until it was time to pick him up.

Mr. Dubinion had worked more than thirty years for the Midline Railroad, but because of his kidney failure, had taken early retirement. He had minimal benefits under the Railroad Retirement Program. Dialysis equipment and supplies were not covered.

Like Wayne Willis, he was laid back and easy going—not ruffled easily. He had accepted his kidney failure with equanimity. A quiet spoken member of the Second Presbyterian Church of the Redeemer, he never seemed to question that he had been dealt any bad cards in life. Perhaps, predestination influences from his religious upbringing precluded any complaints.

When he had been dialyzing for a little over two months, he started home training. I knew training Mrs. Dubinion wasn't going to be easy, but the options were few. It was time to begin.

Mrs. Dubinion was afraid of machines in general. And, I thought, dialysis machines, with her husband's blood visibly flowing through the tubing, would petrify her. Before even suggesting she start training, I wanted to acclimate her to the dialysis room and get her accustomed to watching the procedure.

Her first day of observation began with a vociferous cry. "Good heavens, Dr. Van Giesen! I get so nauseous when I see Howard's blood going through those tubes. I don't think I can sit here and watch any of this."

I had just left the dialysis room, and was about to make rounds at University when I heard her outcry. I rushed back to the dialysis room and found Mrs. Dubinion in her chair with her knees against her chest, her eyes tightly shut and her head buried in the pillow on which she'd been sitting.

She remained in this position for several minutes. When she removed the pillow and looked at Howard attached to the dialysis machine, she became nauseated. "I'm going to throw up. Quick, give me a bucket or something!"

Mrs. Harrison grabbed an emesis basin and eased it onto Mrs. Dubinion's lap just in time. After the nausea and vomiting abated, I spoke to Mrs. Dubinion, offered her sips of ginger ale, and very softly, suggested that she come with me to the break room and lie down for a while. She stayed there until her husband finished dialysis. She had recovered enough by then to drive him home.

Events progressed slowly after Mrs. Dubinion's initial encounter with dialysis. Mr. Dubinion continued to tolerate dialysis without complaining and his blood work showed modest improvement. Mrs. Dubinion, on the other hand, found it continually difficult to look at blood in the lines. I was seriously concerned that maybe, after all, she wasn't going to be able to learn enough about dialysis to safely dialyze her husband.

Mrs. Harrison organized a training manual for Mrs. Dubinion. She drew pictures of the steps necessary for proper dialysis technique and began going over them with her each dialysis day.

A month later, Mrs. Dubinion was still unable to sit and watch her husband being dialyzed. She complained of nausea regularly, and kept the emesis basin in her lap. However, the spells were less frequent and didn't last as long. Three months into the training, she felt comfortable enough to sit and watch without the emesis basin. This was a major accomplishment on their journey to home dialysis; but Mrs. Dubinion, was still a long way from becoming a trusted dialysis partner.

Finally, I think Mrs. Dubinion came to understand and accept that we were really serious about getting her husband home and safely on dialysis. We weren't to be dissuaded.

I was beginning to feel a little pressure to move Howard Dubinion home, in order to open up his spot for others. Several patients with chronic renal failure were on the Harper Street clinic waiting list, while their doctors, in neighboring South Carolina, were managing them with Giovannetti style diets. I had been on Harper Street for almost two years. During that time, we had been able to train the Willises for home dialysis, Robert Jackson was now a self-care, out of hospital, dialysis patient, and we were making every effort to send the Dubinions home to dialyze.

Word had spread in the medical community that I was accepting older patients for hemodialysis and training them for home dialysis. I was keeping a list of patients that referring physicians deemed possible candidates. I needed more space to dialyze, if I was to take on additional patients.

IN DECEMBER 1970, I made the move to a larger office in the same vicinity, near to the two hospitals with which I was primarily associated. The new office was on 15th Street and considerably larger than the one on Harper. There was a large room for three dialysis machines. I continued using my Maytag and obtained two used Travenol machines — updated models with their own roller pumps. I continued using the SigmaMotor pump with my Maytag.

CHAPTER 25

NEW DIALYSIS CRITERIA

God Works in a Mysterious Way.
Christian Hymn by William Cowper, 1793

Soon, all spots in the new dialysis quarters would be filled. I'd hired additional nursing staff. The nurse to patient ratio was 1:1 — ideal for home training. Home dialysis, I felt, was the intermediate goal, but when transplantation wasn't an option, it was the final goal.

I didn't have strict criteria for accepting patients for dialysis. I tried to keep an open mind. Most dialysis facilities, during this era, were not dialyzing diabetic patients. Patients over the age of sixty were generally not considered candidates. Children were not routinely dialyzed, nor were patients with significant heart disease. Not only were these exclusions for chronic dialysis understood in the fledgling dialysis community, but physicians, generally, were not referring these patients for dialysis.

I was surprised when I received a call from Dr. Jim Woodstock, a general practitioner in rural Richmond County, asking me to see Rudy Fleming in consultation. Rudy, a long time friend of Jim, and pastor at Groves New Eden Baptist Church, was a Type one Diabetic.

Jim told me he had been following Rudy for many years, that his diabetes was exceptionally well controlled on long acting insulin, and that he was "as fine a person as you would ever want to meet."

"George," he said, "Rudy's going blind and recently his creatinine and BUN have started rising significantly. He's had diabetes since the age of about ten. Seems the diabetes is finally taking its toll. I'm hoping you will take a look at him and give me your thoughts about offering him dialysis."

"I'll be glad to see him, Jim, but from what you've told me already, I suspect I'll not recommend dialysis," I said.

"Well, I'd appreciate you seeing him anyway."

Rudy Fleming, LLD, arrived at my office with his wife, Effie, on a beautiful, cool, autumn afternoon. He was using a cane and holding on to his wife's arm as he entered. He was wearing dark glasses, which he didn't remove as he sat in the waiting room.

They were right on time for their appointment, which I fit in fifteen minutes before my regularly scheduled patients were to arrive. Rudy, at a little less than six feet tall, with coal black hair parted down the middle, was forty-five years old. He didn't look like a patient with chronic renal failure. His color was good. He walked erect, even while resting his hand on his wife's arm. They were ushered into my office and sat on the sofa across from my desk.

"Doctor," he began in a deep baritone voice. "Thank you very much for working us into your heavy schedule. Jim Woodstock speaks highly of you. I'll try not to take up too much of your time."

"Well, I've known Jim since we both were in medical school. A good friend and an excellent doctor," I replied.

"You see, Doctor, I've had diabetes for as long as I can remember. But I never let it hold me back. That is, until my vision started going bad about a year ago. Jim sent me to Dr. Bartholomew, Jim's own ophthalmologist, and he's been following me since. I've been told there's little that can be done for my eyes. He's already classified me as legally blind.

"Doctor Van Giesen, Jim says that my kidneys are failing. I still feel I have a lot of work to do in the name of the Lord. I want to keep going as long as I feel good enough and capable of doing God's will. I've never had any serious problems in keeping my diabetes under control. Effie has seen to it that I always have the proper diet, and I've established a work relaxation regimen that allows me to stay mentally healthy, and emotionally and physically strong."

The reverend was delivering me a synoptic rendition of his medical history without my asking him one question. I just listened.

He continued. "About a year ago, Jim had mentioned to me that he was a little worried about some changes in my blood work that indicated my kidneys were not working as well as they should. A week or so ago, he called me at home and said he wanted me to see you. I asked him, at the time, if my kidneys were giving out on me. He just said that, well, they were weakening.

"You see, Doctor, I've read a lot about my burden. I know pretty much about the course of long-standing diabetes. I know the different body systems eventually break down. And like I said, I've got a lot more work that I really need to get done before I become invalided."

I could see he was beginning to visualize his diabetes stopping him from doing everything he wanted to do. It was evident he wasn't ready for that to happen.

"Doctor, you see, my vision hasn't slowed me down. I'm able to attend to the needs of my parishioners. I still make hospital rounds. I still make house calls. I preach at funerals. I still attend meetings after meetings about church matters. There are good people in my church. I've never had to ask for help. These good people are there to help before I have to ask. Good people, Doctor. A blessing from God, I call it.

"I'm still able to deliver sermons. I need help getting to and from the pulpit, but once there, I'm as good as I've ever been. I can't see individuals in the congregation—it's all a blur. I've never used notes when preaching, so not having vision hasn't affected the quality of my sermons," he chuckled slightly. "At least, no one has told me my vigor has gone," he smiled broadly.

I wanted to hear more from the Reverend Fleming, but I needed to get to my other afternoon appointments. "Reverend," I said, "I want to get started with your evaluation right away. The quickest and easiest way is for you to be admitted. If I can get a room in University, will you be able to go today?"

"Yes," he said. "I'm ready to do what's necessary."

In the hospital, I was able to elicit symptoms of uremia that the reverend had not alluded to in my office. I was unsure if he was trying to keep his symptoms from his wife, or if he was such a stoic person that he refused to acknowledge his condition.

He told me his appetite had been off for the last six months, at least. His unfailing stamina was not as unfailing as he had suggested earlier. He frequently found the need for afternoon naps to "reinvigorate" himself. And finally, he was having increasingly frequent episodes of nausea.

On physical examination, his blood pressure was elevated. He showed evidence of an enlarged heart, and he was beginning to accumulate excess fluid as shown by edema of the feet. His twenty-four hour creatinine clearances confirmed that, in fact, he had end stage renal disease — secondary to diabetic nephropathy. He needed dialysis. It could be postponed a bit. However, except for being a diabetic, he surely fit the criteria for dialysis. Was he a candidate for home training? Without talking to him or his wife, I couldn't say. Would dialyzing a diabetic be in the patient's best interest? I wasn't sure. It was too early in the new field of chronic dialysis to know. Reverend Fleming's courage and determination to pursue his goals inspired me. I wanted to offer him a spot on dialysis.

Jerry Farmer, a deacon at New Eden, was one of a number of church members to contact me. He wanted me to know more about his pastor, he said. "He's a real devotee to the game of golf. I've played golf with him for the last ten years — every Wednesday afternoon. When his eyes began deceiving him, and he had trouble seeing the ball on the tee, he would ask me to line him up straight in the direction I thought the ball should go. Then he'd ask me to place the face of his club next to the ball. He'd take a back swing, then let it go. The first time he did this, the ball went straight down the fairway about two hundred yards. I couldn't believe it. But now I've seen it happen this way so many times I don't even think about him not being able to see the ball on the tee or in the air. It's pretty impressive." He hesitated a moment then added, "Rudy Fleming's a remarkable individual, Doctor. He's inspirits me and all those who know him. When he sets his mind to something, there's no stopping him. We still play golf every Wednesday."

After hearing from several of his parishioners over the next few weeks, I knew I'd find a place for him to dialyze in our clinic, and that he would be a good risk for home training. I was prepared to offer him the last spot on the Monday, Wednesday, Friday schedule, if he was willing to be trained for home dialysis.

CHAPTER 26

HOME TRAINING

Time to fish or cut bait.
Common English Colloquial Expression

The Dubinions were still training to dialyze at home. Since moving to the larger office, we had been able to put Mr. Dubinion on a Monday, Wednesday, Friday schedule. The training was proceeding a little better in the new environment. The nurses and I had gone over and over everything that must be done to insure their safety.

Although Mrs. Dubinion still had reservations about her ability "to dialyze alone," as she put it, there was little more we could do to bolster her confidence. I reminded her, we were all confident she would know exactly what to do if a line came unconnected, a coil leaked, or in the worst of conditions, a coil burst. If she retained her composure, I assured, she would have no trouble remedying the problem. Hopefully, we would soon be able to find out how well Mrs. Dubinion's training paid off.

There was only one obstacle in the way. The Dubinions did not have a dialysis machine. Earlier in the year their church had raised enough funds to help cover the dialysis supplies — my kidney account helped with the shortfall. Even so, with dialysis machines costing around $3000, the church did not have the financial resources to purchase one for them.

During this period, I learned that General Mills, under the Betty Crocker label, would redeem their coupons for a dialysis machine. Several elders of the church asked me to speak to the congregation about the Betty Crocker program.

One Sunday, after the service was over, Reverend Prichard asked the congregation to remain for a few minutes. He said he had a special announcement to make. He introduced me to the worshippers, and I made my way to the pulpit at his direction. I gave a brief account of the Dubinion's situation and told them about the General Mills Betty Crocker coupon program.

After my talk, coupons from church members and their friends began pouring into the church fund set up for the Dubinions. Soon, word spread into the Dubinion's mobile home park, and in a few weeks, the fund had over 35,000 coupons, then 100,000, and in four months, more than 500,000, enough to purchase a Travenol machine.

We accompanied the Dubinions to their trailer to help them decide where to locate their new machine. The trailer was a double wide manufactured by Clanton Homes. There was ample space for the Travenol, which they decided to put in the second bedroom, next to the bathroom.

Within a week, the Dubinions were dialyzing at home. As with the Willises, we stayed with them until we, and they, were satisfied that all was well. And though my phone rang regularly for the first two weeks of their dialyzing at home, Mrs. Dubinion proved to be up to the task. There were no real problems, just minor issues with which she still needed reassurance.

Within a month of home dialyses, the Dubinions settled into a regular routine. The telephone calls were less frequent, then finally ceased. The shunt continued to function and the dialyses ran smoothly as Mrs. Dubinion, though still stressed with the responsibility, developed more confidence. Since their insurance policies didn't cover dialysis, the Dubinions depended on funds raised by their church to purchase dialysis supplies.

Mr. Dubinion thrived on dialysis for a while. He regained much of his strength and took up one of his old hobbies again. He and several buddies met every two weeks to fish at Clark Hill, a short distance from Augusta.

Mrs. Dubinion kept her job at Segars. Surprisingly, working full time there and then coming home to dialyze Howard in the evening worked well for them. She said that Howard took more responsibility for the home now that she had two full time jobs.

CHAPTER 27

A VACATION SHORTENED

"Any problems that may occur have ultimately been caused by you, because you are responsible for where you are and what you are doing there." **Garth Stein; A novel; The Art of Racing in the Rain published by Harper Collins 2008**

My practice had become less a general medical and more of a practice for a specialized kidney disease. At times, I had too many patients requiring peritoneal or hemodialysis. I couldn't expect the three other doctors in my call group, internists, to manage my patients' dialysis needs when I wasn't on call. I needed someone to share calls, someone experienced in dialytic procedures.

An incident that happened to me one summer weekend when I was not on call, and out of town, confirmed this necessity. With my weekend off, my family and I had driven to Fripp Island, on the South Carolina coast, for a few days of rest and relaxation. I was in a small bateau, casting for shrimp in the canal behind the house in which we were staying. I heard a siren blaring from a distance down the single road leading to the south end of the island. It stopped in front of our house. My wife was standing on the front porch balcony, awestruck. A young man wearing a red cap and in fireman's garb, jumped from his truck with a megaphone in his hand. "Do you know where your husband is?" he asked excitedly.

She pointed to the canal in the back. "What's this all about?" she insisted.

"It's an emergency — about one of his patients in Augusta, ma'am." Then he ran to the dock behind the house and began shouting through the megaphone, "Dr. Van Giesen, Dr. George Van Giesen. This is an emergency. Please return to your dock. Return to your dock. Now!"

I was so deep in the marsh he didn't see me initially, but I clearly heard him. I didn't have a motor on my boat, and it took me about ten minutes to get back to the dock. When he saw me waving my hand and rowing back as fast as I could, he stopped calling.

The man was a member of the Fripp Island Volunteer Fire Department. He had received a call from Janet, my "Jill of all trades." Dr. Jim Taylor, who was taking call for our group, had been summoned to the University Hospital ER to see Julia Kanovich, the last patient I still had on an intermittent peritoneal dialysis program.

Since there was no telephone service at the house, I asked the fireman if I could ride with him and use the phone in his office. I reached Jim, who was still in the ER with Mrs. Kanovich. He told me that she was obviously fluid overloaded and was having some mild, difficulty breathing. He said her electrolytes were okay, she wasn't in any acute danger and just needed a dialysis, he thought.

I knew Jim didn't do peritoneal dialysis. I felt guilty that he was in the position he found himself. I felt guilty for Mrs. Kanovich's situation. I felt a keen sense of responsibility for her. I had started her on peritoneals; now she needed one and I wasn't there to start it. She trusted me to be there, and I felt I had let her down.

I discussed the situation with Jim. This was a Sunday and I had planned to return to Augusta early Monday morning. Jim said he thought Mrs. Kanovich "would hold" until I could start the peritoneal Monday. And she probably could, I told myself. Even so, I made the decision to leave Fripp as soon as I could pack my suitcase.

I was back in Augusta in less than three hours. I went straight to University, and started the dialysis that evening. With removal of the excess fluid, Mrs. Kanovich felt considerably better. So did I.

Not long after the incident on Fripp Island, Dr. Hy Sussman, a good friend and colleague in the Renal section at MCG, joined me in private practice. I had been after Hy to enter practice with me for sometime, and was pleased and gratified when he decided to make the transition. Now, the two of us shared calls and office space. With Hy taking my calls when I was off, I knew my patients were in excellent hands and that no aspects of their care would be left unattended.

JULIA KANOVICH was the last of my chronic peritoneal dialysis patients to make the transition to hemodialysis. With the Dubinions successfully dialyzing at home, a spot was available for her.

Julia, now almost fifty years old, had tolerated her low protein diet and intermittent peritoneal dialysis extremely well over the last two years. She and her husband, Bill, lived in a comfortable home on Augusta's west side. Bill was the chief financial officer for Southbrook Industries, a company involved in managing real estate, among other ventures.

Julia was a thin woman of medium height. In spite of having been on a special diet and intermittent peritoneal dialysis, she prided herself in keeping up appearances. Her gray-streaked hair was cut stylishly short. She always wore nice outfits and had makeup on when coming for dialysis.

She had a pleasant disposition and smiled easily. But she didn't like the fact that she had "this kidney disability." In truth, she resented it highly. She knew I wanted to start her on hemodialysis as soon as we had enough staff and the space for her. She had always been active physically, playing tennis, swimming, and going to the gym. Since being on peritoneal dialysis she had to curtail much of her routine.

I arranged for her to have an AV fistula created several months before she was scheduled to start hemo. I was optimistic about her and her husband being able to learn the skill of venipuncture as well as learning the intricacies of performing dialysis at home. By the time she started, the fistula had matured. It remained patent (open) throughout the time she was on dialysis.

We had discussed home dialysis a number of times. At first, she did not embrace the idea. She and Bill had two teenage daughters, and Julia was concerned as to how her children might be adversely affected by the introduction of an artificial kidney into their home.

I made arrangements for her and Bill to visit with the Willises. After witnessing them dialyze in their home, both she and Bill felt much more comfortable about the procedure.

The insurance that Bill's company provided had covered Julia's peritoneal dialyses. Of course, these treatments were performed in the hospital. I was unsure as to whether hemodialysis procedures, in an outpatient facility, would be covered.

I had an opportunity to talk with their insurance agent before Julia began her treatments. I asked if outpatient dialysis was a treatment modality they recognized and would cover. Since Bill had asked him this same question earlier, he had a ready answer. The major medical section of their policy covered doctors' office visits. The policy did not have in place a payment schedule specifically for hemodialysis. But the number of office visits was not limited. The agent felt that if bills were presented as office visits, not hemodialysis treatments, reimbursement would be made.

Each month, as long as she was dialyzing in the office, I sent my charge, ten dollars, to the insurance company. Their insurance company continued to pay for the procedure throughout the time Julia was in training. Major medical provisions in their policy allowed them to purchase a Travenol machine. After she began home dialysis, necessary supplies also continued to be covered.

Bill was the responsible dialysis partner, but Julia wanted to learn how to insert the needles in her fistula. She and Bill both became skilled venipuncturists. Gaining vascular access was never a problem for the Kanovichs. They were trained for home dialysis in four months.

CHAPTER 28

CENTER OR HOME DIALYSIS

"Five patients with previous experience of home dialysis ... had internal arteriovenous fistulae created... After training of the spouses or patients to insert the needles ... the patients (were) maintained on fistula dialysis in the home ... The safe use of a blood pump in the home, overnight, was achieved by the addition of an extra monitor on the outflow (arterial) blood line." **Stanley Shaldon and Sheila McKay - Use of Internal Arteriovenous Fistula in Home Dialysis Br. Med. J. 1968 Dec 14; 4(5632): 671-673**

The early seventies saw an expansion of chronic dialysis facilities, throughout this country and abroad. Financing the establishment and maintenance of dialysis centers had long been an obstacle to taking care of the increasing number of patients needing long-term dialysis.

When Belding Scribner dialyzed his first (chronic) patient in the spring of 1960, he had obtained a grant from the National Institutes of Health. Later, he received additional support from the Hartford Foundation.

THE HARTFORD FOUNDATION was established in 1929 by two brothers, John and George Hartford, President and CEO respectively of the Great Atlantic and Pacific Tea

Co (A&P Supermarkets). Until the 1970s, when the National Institutes of Health began increasing their funding, the Hartford Foundation was one of the largest contributors to medical research in this country.

MANY INSURANCE COMPANIES remained reluctant to cover costs for chronic dialysis. Funding became difficult to obtain and many centers turned to home dialysis. The percentages of patients dialyzing at home and those in-center varied greatly center to center. For example, at one time in the state of Washington, a large majority of patients were dialyzing at home. In other facilities, all patients were being dialyzed in-center.

My approach to dialysis remained the same. I wanted to train all my patients to dialyze at home. Even though I had accepted the Reverend Fleming, a diabetic, I had no other chronic diabetic renal patients referred to me for several years. Referring physicians were still reluctant to suggest dialysis to their diabetic patients at that time.

We had begun dialyzing five days a week soon after we moved from our Harper Street clinic to the larger building on 15th Street, but I did not want to go to a six-day schedule. Chronic dialysis had not become a business, at least to me. It was just a large part of my practice.

Each morning, Monday through Friday, I made rounds on each patient in our dialysis room before I rounded at the hospitals. All of our center dialysis patients now had AV fistulas — Mr. Dubinion, at home, still had his shunt. In the beginning, I inserted all the needles in the patients' vessels, started the dialysis, and waited until all patients were stable before I left.

Over the next year and a half, our dialysis team, maintained five patients on dialysis — three on a Monday, Wednesday, Friday schedule, and two on a Tuesday, Thursday schedule.

Wilma Walker, a retired schoolteacher from Lucy Laney High School, had a policy from Richmond County School District that might have allowed her to train for home dialysis. But, she lived in an apartment complex by herself. She remained an in-center patient.

Beulah Helmly was nineteen and had just graduated from Laney High School. She lived at home with her invalid mother and a younger sister. They had no insurance. The family was on welfare. Home dialysis was out.

Ola June Watson, a thirty-year-old former maid at the Richmond Hotel, hadn't been able to work for the last year because of failing kidneys. She too was on welfare and lived alone.

The Reverend Fleming had begun dialysis and I hoped he would be able to dialyze at home. And finally, there was Robert Jackson, who, I was hoping, would be accepted on a transplant program soon.

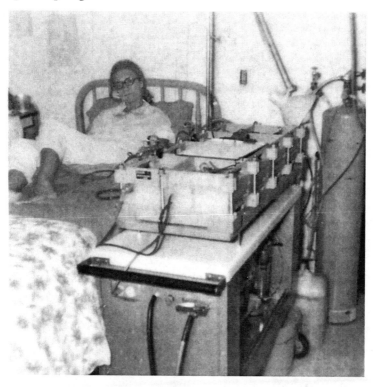

One of the first home dialysis patients, Nancy Spaeth (1968), Seattle, hooked to a flat plate dialyzer (Photo courtesy Nancy Spaeth)

CHAPTER 29

CONSULTATIONS

Library Dedication pays Tribute to pathologist.
The D. Frank Mullins, Jr. Library will be a lasting tribute to a doctor who devoted so much of his own time to giving information.
Toni Baker Tuesday, April 8, 1987, THE BEEPER

Most of my chronic renal failure patients came to my office. On occasions, I would make trips to surrounding counties to see them in consultation.

D. Frank Mullins, M.D., a member of the clinical faculty at MCG, had an independent pathology practice in Augusta. He had established the Mullins Pathology and Cytology Laboratory of Augusta in the 1950s. His practice centered around his lab, but he also had a consulting practice in a number of small town hospitals and clinics, in both Georgia and South Carolina. His visits helped these small facilities maintain their accreditation, and provided a greater number of laboratory services for their patients.

Frank owned a small plane in which he flew to these, out of the way places, on a regular basis. On times, he would ask me to go with him, especially when the local doctors had patients with kidney problems that raised questions about dialysis.

On one of our visits, in the early fall of 1971, we were to meet Dr. Campbell Dixon at a small hospital across the Savannah River, in Jasper County. Dr. Dixon was the only physician practicing there at the time. Frank and I were met by the doctor's receptionist/nurse, Sarah, at the small, unpaved landing field a few miles from the hospital, which Dr. Dixon's father had established in the late 1920s. She took us to Dykes restaurant, the only one in town. It was patronized by the Kiwanians and the Rotarians, and noted for home cooked Southern food.

After our lunch of sweet potatoes, rice, cornbread, and fried chicken, Sarah drove us to the clinic, attached by a walkway to the 30-bed hospital. Sarah handed me a list of patients Dr. Dixon wanted me to see. Rarely did I meet with Dr. Dixon. Usually, he was too busy in the hospital, operating, or making rounds.

The list included several patients with albumin in the urine, and one, a forty-year-old dairy farmer, Sam Attaling, who was clinically, and by lab results, severely uremic. I felt sure Mr. Attaling had chronic renal failure secondary to longstanding glomerular nephritis. After examining the other patients, I made notes on all their charts as Dr. Dixon had requested.

My recommendation for Sam Attaling with uremia was, "he needs dialysis as soon as possible." Also, I noted that I would be glad to make arrangements for him to be hospitalized in Augusta as soon as I returned.

When Frank and I had finished our work, and the last clinic patient had gone, Sarah drove us to the airport and we flew back to Augusta in clear weather under a waning August moon.

I heard no more from Dr. Dixon until Frank and I returned six weeks later. There was another list of patients for me to see. Sam's name wasn't on the list. I asked Sarah what had happened to him. She told me, "Dr. Dixon bought an artificial kidney, put a shunt in Sam's arm, and started dialyzing him, as you suggested."

I was a little befuddled when she explained this to me. I knew Dr. Dixon had no experience in dialysis and I assumed neither had she. She said a manual came with the machine and that she and Dr. Dixon read through it and felt that they could perform the treatment themselves. She took me to the room they used for dialysis. The machine was still there. It was the same model as the Travenol machines I was using in Augusta.

Sarah went on to explain that Dr. Dixon placed a shunt in Sam's arm and dialyzed him twice. She said neither of the dialysis treatments seemed to relieve his symptoms. "He didn't come back for his third treatment. We called his home and spoke with his wife. She explained that Sam didn't want any more treatments. Several days later, she called the office and told us Sam died in his sleep."

I flew with Frank to other small hospitals over the next several years to see patients in consultation, but Dr. Dixon quit leaving lists of patients to be seen—for what reason I never knew.

Tragically, in February 1973, Frank Mullins died of a crash in his own plane near Greer, SC on a trip to the hospital there.

CHAPTER 30

DOCTORS HOSPITAL

*"Grand opening ceremonies for Doctors Hospital of Augusta takes place the weekend Nov 2-4." **Augusta Chronicle Nov 4, 1973***

The new Doctors Hospital opened in early November 1973. Construction of the adjacent Professional Building had begun. I added my name to the list of doctors who planned to move their practices here.

Initially, my thoughts were to have a small dialysis room connected to my office, a room in which I would continue to dialyze, and train patients and their families for home dialysis. I had given little thought to expanding our dialysis capabilities.

Over the last several years, I had been extremely busy, seeing up to thirty patients a day in my office, and making rounds in three hospitals. Also, I was attending regular meetings with the new Doctors Hospital Board of Directors.

The Federal government, following the passage of the National End Stage Renal Disease (ESRD) Program in 1972, determined that the best way of ensuring adequate delivery of medical care to patients needing dialysis was to set up networks organized geographically. Originally, 32 service areas were created nationwide. Later, in 1987, the 32 areas were reduced to 18. Each network included representatives of the federally approved treatment facilities in the region, along with patients and professionals involved directly in the care of patients. The record showed that, originally, we had been approved for three dialysis stations.

As the Federal Medicare ESRD program was being cranked up, facilities that had been functioning under earlier guidelines were advised to notify the authorities as to the number of dialysis stations they would need as the new regulations became effective in July 1973.

In working on the application for approval of the new dialysis facility at Doctors Hospital, I planned to ask for approval of three stations for dialysis. But, the number of patients on my waiting list was increasing. As we filled out the application forms, Janet, my office/dialysis assistant, suggested, "Why don't we ask for approval for ten stations? I think it would be easier to get approval for more stations now, than later."

I told her I didn't have a problem requesting more stations, but I thought it would take us a long time before we would fill all those additional spots." On the form, however, I asked for ten and we were approved.

I significantly underestimated the growing demand for dialysis services. When the Federal program for ESRD was implemented, chronic dialysis took on a new life. The selection committees were fazed out. Diabetics were accepted for dialysis. Elderly patients were given a second chance for life. Almost any patient with chronic progressive renal failure was a candidate for dialysis now.

I was impressed how quickly my list of patients with this diagnosis—ESRD—grew. By the time the new Professional building at Doctors Hospital was completed, I had enough patients on the list to fill the new ten-station dialysis facility immediately. And that included dialyzing six days a week.

My new office and dialysis clinic were ready for occupancy in late 1973. I moved there in February 1974. I traded in my used Travenol machines for ten new Travenol RSP machines.

I put the Maytag machine in storage and had planned to keep it, for sentimental reasons. Unfortunately, it was discarded inadvertently during one of my family's many moves.

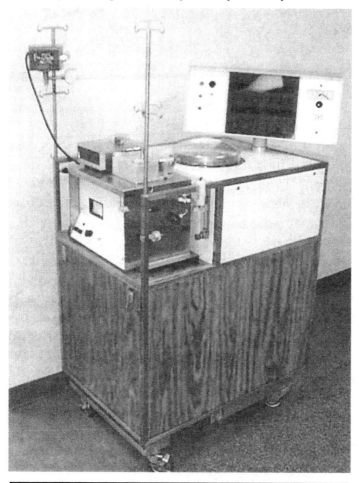

Travenol RSP dialysis machine, same model as those in new dialysis center near Doctors Hospital.

The new dialysis center was attached to my office, with a short hall connecting the two units. As of July 1, 1973, the Federal government was picking up the tab for practically all patients needing chronic dialysis. The main impediment—financial—to treating patients with chronic renal failure had been removed.

My emphasis on training patients for home dialysis remained a priority as Augusta Dialysis Center transitioned from a three-station dialysis clinic to the ten-station facility in the professional building across from Doctors Hospital. We continued to maintain a home training room, along with a self-dialysis section—for those patients who wanted to dialyze themselves and to set their own schedules—for as long as I was in practice.

THE REVEREND FLEMING already had started home training before we moved. Those sessions were put on hold when he suffered a massive heart attack six weeks after beginning dialysis. We continued to dialyze him in the hospital while he was being managed for his cardiac condition. As might be expected, his condition only worsened. He never recovered. Slowly, and tragically, his life ebbed away. He never regained enough cardiac function to sustain life.

Robert Jackson continued in-center dialysis on a completely independent program. We set aside a corner spot for Robert, where he was allowed to dialyze on his own schedule. On the days he wasn't dialyzing, he was given a paying job as a dialysis assistant and worked with the nurses participating in all aspects of dialysis.

Robert's blood pressure was never satisfactorily controlled in spite of tight fluid regulation and potent antihypertensives. When he began having severe headaches again, and his ophthalmologist found worsening of his eye grounds, I asked Robert to stop by my office and told him of the need for surgery, to remove his kidneys—a drastic procedure, but one I, along with several other physicians felt was necessary.

Robert, never one to complain about anything, said he was willing to go along with our recommendation. He said he understood the implications of doing nothing. He underwent the surgical procedure without complications. Having the surgery proved to have been the correct decision. His blood pressure dropped to safe levels with minimal drug support, his headaches subsided, his vision improved, and in spite of persistently lower Hgb levels, his sense of well being greatly improved.

Robert continued working in the clinic and took on another job. When a friend of mine, a physician who developed seizures, was forced to give up driving his car; Robert became his driver for a number of years until he was called for his cadaver transplant.

His transplant worked well for many years. Eventually, Robert developed a cardiomyopathy and after a series of hospitalizations succumbed to his heart failure. He was thirty-five years old.

Julia Kanovich struggled with home dialysis. It interfered with her social life. Although she had adapted to giving up most of the physical activities she had enjoyed prior to her kidney failure, she still liked to play canasta with her friends. She still wanted to be more involved with her church guild. She liked to dress up and go out for lunch with her two girls, but she complained, "dialysis always seems to be in the way."

Dialysis was a burden she never was able to unload. In the mid '70s, she received a cadaver transplant. It functioned well. She had begun to "feel almost human again" following the transplant. For a number of years life was good, but in the late '70s, she began having severe anginal attacks. Her cardiovascular disease progressed rapidly and she suffered a fatal myocardial infarction in the summer of 1979. She was fifty-eight years old.

Howard Dubinion and his wife began home dialysis in 1971, acquiring their dialysis machine only months before the Betty Crocker coupon exchange for artificial kidneys program was discontinued. Although the Dubinions' home dialysis went well for the first two years, unfortunately Mr. Dubinion succumbed to a dreaded complication of dialysis. He developed a skin condition with multiple painful ulcerations accompanied by severe infections—a condition called Calciphylaxis, for which no successful therapy was available. After repeated hospitalizations, he died in early 1974 at the age of sixty-two.

Wayne Willis, who went home to dialyze on the machine of his own design, continued to dialyze on it for many years. He remained employed at McDougall Industries, fitting dialysis into his schedule so it didn't interfere with his work. In the late '80s, he received a successful transplant from his brother. His health began failing several years later. Complications from severe cardiovascular disease ensued and he died following repeated hospitalizations in 1990. He was sixty-nine years old.

CHAPTER 31

THE CHANGE

Sec 405.2101 Objectives of the end-stage renal disease (ESRD) program

1. To assist beneficiaries who have been diagnosed as having ESRD to receive the care they need.
2. To encourage proper distribution and effective utilization of ESRD treatment resources while maintaining or improving quality of care.
3. To provide the flexibility necessary for the efficient delivery of appropriate care by physicians and facilities; and
4. To encourage self-dialysis or transplantation for the maximum practical number of patients who are medically, socially, and psychologically suitable for such treatment.

In the decade or so prior to 1973, a modest number of patients with chronic renal failure were fortunate enough to have their lives extended by dialysis. But, during this era, a far greater number of patients were not afforded that opportunity. Some estimates suggest that those not receiving dialysis was three to four times as great as those receiving it.

Before July 1973, a large majority of patients with chronic renal failure were dialyzing at home. By July 1974, one year after the Federal program began, over 40,000 patients were being dialyzed, but less than half of those patients were on home dialysis. The increase in outpatient dialysis centers, both non and for-profit, lessened the urgency of physicians and patients to opt for home dialysis. Center dialysis was easier for most patients and physicians. Although there are more than 700,000 patients being dialyzed in this country, less than 14,000 of them are home based as of this writing.

The Federal ESRD program, beginning in 1973, rendered the ad hoc approach to treating chronic renal failure obsolete. There were many failings of that earlier era, not the least of which was refusing patients treatment because of their lack of money or lack of worth. But, the offering of choices to patients whose options were so few, gave hope, encouragement, and opportunity to some patients for a second chance at life.

The vision, determination, and tenacity of the early pioneers in dialysis and renal transplantation paved the way for multitudes to benefit from these new disciplines. If the present system of delivering care to patients with chronic renal failure had been in place in those earlier days, the lives of Jimmy Wells and Rita Kimble, along with thousands of others who never gained access to the system, would have played out much differently.

I am privileged to have been practicing medicine during a time when chronic dialysis and renal transplantation were in their infancy. It is satisfying to know that, in this country, patients with Bright's Disease, Chronic Progressive Renal Failure, or ESRD, whatever name it is called, are no longer alone in shouldering the financial burden for the treatment of their condition. Thanks to the dedicated physicians, patients, and public servants who labored long for the passage of Public Law 92-603, *this* onus has been removed.

In the era before Renal Medicare, dialysis for chronic renal failure was a hands-on procedure, requiring the cooperation and interaction of patients, doctors, nurses, technicians, dietitians, social workers, and family. Although, Chronic

Dialysis in 2016 is more technically intricate than it was in 1970, its success relies on these very same interpersonal dependences — now as much as then.

NOTES TO CHAPTERS

Chapter 1

In 1967, the President's Office of Science and Technology established a committee of experts to study and evaluate all aspects of chronic kidney disease. Carl Gottschalk, M.D., a Nephrologist at the University of North Carolina, chaired this committee.

The committee determined that two recently established treatment modalities for chronic kidney failure, dialysis, and transplantation were no longer considered experimental. Because of the expense and the almost universal lack of insurance coverage for these procedures, the committee recommended a Federal program under Medicare cover these forms of treatment.

Their recommendations were shelved for several years. Robert A. Rettig, PhD, a member of the National Academy of Sciences, has written extensively on the origins of the Social Security amendments of 1972. His very interesting and thorough account of how this legislation, and particularly the legislation providing Medicare coverage for chronic renal failure (Section 2991 of Public Law 92-603) came into being, can be found in **Biomedical Politics 1991, Kathi E. Hanna, Editor; Pages 176-214.**

Chapter 2

Prologue Magazine; Summer 2004 issue, Volume 36 #2, printed quarterly by the National Archives and Records Administration, details Lyndon Johnson's masterful political maneuvering, leading up to the passage of the Civil Rights Law (Public Law 88-352) in 1964.

δ

A brief biography of Roy Harris, by Christopher A. Huff, can be found in *New Georgia Encyclopedia, January 10, 2014.*

Chapter 3

Sergio Giovannetti, the Italian Nephrologist who, in the early 1960s, studied the effects of an ultra low protein diet on chronic renal failure, defines Uremia as "a battery of signs and symptoms caused by renal failure." He describes three different groups of "uremic manifestations—those that are easily corrected by dialysis—for example: nausea, vomiting, anorexia." A second group "caused by overhydration —high blood pressure, edema, dyspnea" being examples, "treated by removal of excess fluid via dialytic methods." And third, a group of signs and symptoms, "anemia, pruritus, certain hormonal and metabolic abnormalities" being examples, "not directly affected by dialysis." *Nutritional Treatment of Chronic Renal Failure, 1989: Ed. S. Giovannetti; chapter 5, p 29-32*

Chapter 4

Richard Bright published four clinical writings on kidney disease. In 1827, the first of these writings appeared in *Volume I* of his *Medical Reports*. None of these are still in print. In 1937, Dr. A. Arnold Osman edited *The Original Papers of Richard Bright on Renal Disease*, published by *Oxford University Press, London,* in which are included all of Bright's publications on diseases of the kidneys. *Volume I* of *Medical Reports* is the most famous of Bright's publications on kidney disease. This section deals with 24 cases "Illustrative of some of the appearances observable on the examination of diseases terminating in dropsical effusion" (a condition in which the serous fluids accumulate in body cavities or in bodily tissues; pericarditis, ascites, and peripheral edema being examples.)

δ

J. Stewart Cameron, in *Nephrology, Dialysis and Transplantation, 1997; 12; p 1526-1539,* points out that Osman was one of the first physicians to focus his study and medical practice on kidney disease. He established the first Nephritis Clinic at Guy's Hospital in 1930 and "almost certainly was the first physician to call himself a 'nephrologist.'"

δ

The book by Diana Berry and Campbell Mackenzie, *Richard Bright 1789-1858; Physician in an Age of Revolution and Reform; Royal Society of Medicine Limited; 1992* presents a very complete and interestingly written account of Dr. Bright's personal and professional life, his travels, his travelogues, his kidney research, and his insights into the connection of dropsy with "coagulable urine and structural changes in the kidneys."

The authors document the dismal therapeutic options available to physicians practicing in those days: purgatives, mercurials along with opium and antimony, counter irritation, leeches, and a wide variety of herbs and minerals among the many other emperic formulations, which were usually applied in a random fashion with little regard as to the specific disease or condition.

The 1959 edition of Cecil and Loeb's, *Textbook of Medicine,* attests that "therapy in uremia is wholly palliative."

δ

Neal Bricker and associates, *American Journal of Medicine, 1960, 28: 77-97*, proposed using the term Chronic Bright's Disease for all chronic renal conditions leading to progressive irreversible failure.

Seldin, Carter, and Rector, *Chapter 5, Consequences of Renal Failure and Their Management, Diseases of the Kidney; Strauss and Welt, 1963*, refer to "all forms of chronic progressive renal pathology" as Chronic Bright's Disease.

Chapter 5

Cohen reported in the *Canadian Medical Association Journal, May 1963*, of his experience with peritoneal dialysis in 14 patients, eight of whom had chronic renal disease. Although only one patient with kidney failure survived longer than 3 months, that patient was still living nine months following her first dialysis. The suggestion was made that peritoneal dialysis should be considered at least once in any patient with chronic renal failure who has become decompensated (from fluid overload, dehydration, worsening of underlying disease, or some other acute condition).

In 1964, Linder and Bottiglier published a case report in the *Archives of Internal Medicine* of a patient with chronic renal failure treated successfully for 12 months with intermittent peritoneal dialysis.

In the same year, Boen, Mion,Curtis, and Shilipetar reported, in the *Transactions of the American Society for Artificial Internal Organs*, the successful treatment of a small number of patients with chronic renal disease, utilizing the intermittent repeated puncture technique for peritoneal dialysis. One of these patients had been treated for 20 months, another for 7 months, and another for 3 months.

Chapter 6

"The main therapeutic measures employed for treating renal patients, including those with chronic renal failure, were, in the past century (19th century), a milk diet and bed rest, both of which were noxious." Sergio Giovannetti reported in *A Historical Review of Low Protein Diets; Nutritional Treatment of Chronic Renal Failure; Springer, 1989.* Dr. Giovannetti references Franz Volhard's experience, in the early 20th century, of relieving uremic symptoms in patients with chronic renal failure after placing them on low protein diets. He points out that, following Volhard's recommendations, most handbooks of kidney disease recommended low protein diets for chronic renal failure, but most did not specify the necessity of supplementing with essential amino acids, or insuring that the proteins were of high biological value.

Little emphasis was placed on altering this approach to the management of chronic renal failure until the mid 1800s *(Biagio Di Iorio, et al; Journal of Nephrology, 26, 143-152 2013)*. These authors point out that Mariano Semmola, while a medical student in Naples, studied the clinical effects on patients with chronic renal failure by varying the protein content in their diets. He concluded that a diet consisting primarily of vegetables (low protein) had the most beneficial effect on kidney function. Sammola published his findings in 1850, in the *Proceedings of the Academy of Naples*.

In his book published in 1885, *Renal Derangements, Lionel S. Beale, M.D. Professor of the Principles and Practice of Medicine and Physician to King's College Hospital, London*, recommended that milk "undoubtedly" should be the "staple article of diet" for patients with chronic renal disease. However, Beale was beginning to recognize the importance of limiting any excess of high protein foods, and meat in particular, which "passes off the body in the form

of urea" and causes extra work for the kidneys "while their
working is seriously impaired."

That changed with the studies of Carmelo Giordano
*(The Use of Exogenous and Endogenouis Urea for Protein
Synthesis in Normal and Uremic Subjects; J Lab Clin Med
62: 1963, 231-235) and later Giovannetti and Maggiore (A
low-nitrogen Diet with Protein of High Biological Value for
Severe Chronic Uremia; Lancet I, p 1000-1004).*

Initial reports (my own experiences included) of the
effectiveness of the Giordano/Giovannetti diet in relieving
the symptoms of uremia were very encouraging. In countries
other than Italy, modifications of the diet were made to satisfy
cultural tastes. Many patients were surviving longer without
uremic symptoms, if they were able to stay on (eat all of) their
diet. But, over the next several years, reports of malnutrition,
severe agitation, bleeding into muscles and subcutaneous
tissues, serum electrolyte disturbances (high potassium
levels), and instances of sudden death were reported.

Chapter 7

In his **Medical Reports**, Dr. Bright expresses his belief that
the failure to find a cure for the disease is due to the fact that
it (Bright's Disease) often is not recognized in its early stages
and by the time it is diagnosed, the damage to the kidneys
are such that no treatment is effective. His admonition to
his fellow clinicians is to be aware of the insidious nature of
"this malady." However, he doubts "whether we have it in
our power, as yet, even at the earliest periods, to destroy the
liability to relapse, or overcome the morbid tendency."

δ

In 1931, Dr. Ralph Falk and Dr. Don Baxter founded Don
Baxter Intravenous Products Corporation. Their aim was to

make intravenous medications and equipment. Dr. Baxter had been a medical missionary in China earlier in his professional life, and in returning to private practice had found that such items were available only in major medical institutions. He believed that ordinary citizens should have access to them as well.

Baxter formed Travenol Laboratories in 1949 as a division of the main company. It was responsible for developing and marketing chemical compounds and medical equipment. In the early 1950s the company collaborated with Dr. Willem Kolff in manufacturing the first commercially built kidney dialysis machine along with the U200A twin coil dialyzer. In 1956, the machine was marketed and sold for $1200. *Modeling and Control of Dialysis Systems, Ed: A.T.Azar; Springer 2013. Baxter Travenol Laboratories, Inc.* (online web site)

Chapter 8

The first successful transplantation of a kidney, from an identical twin to his brother, occurred In Boston in 1954. Other transplants were carried out in Boston and other cities in the ensuing years. Some recipients were given total body radiation. Some were x-irrradiated and given bone marrow infusions. The results of these early treatment protocols were discouraging. Investigators determined that "x-ray as an immunosuppresive agent was too blunt, non specific, and unpredictable." *Renal Transplantation; A Twenty-five Year Experience; Annals of Surgery; 1976 Nov. 184(5) 564-573*

It was not until the early 1960s, when effective immunosuppressive drugs became available, that the modern era for human kidney transplantation began. As Starzl points out in his 1993 manuscript, *The French Heritage in Clinical Kidney Transplantation, Transplant Rev*, "By January 1963 the number of active clinical (transplantation) centers in

America had grown to three --- the Brigham (Boston), the Medical College of Virginia, and the University of Colorado." But, there were two centers in Paris that had "kept the flames (of kidney transplantation) alive" from 1959 through early 1962 when all other efforts were failing." Dr. Starzl, one of the foremost figures in the field of transplantation, attributed much of the success of kidney transplantation to the early efforts of the French pioneers, Drs. Jean Hamburger and Rene Kuss, with their work in Paris.

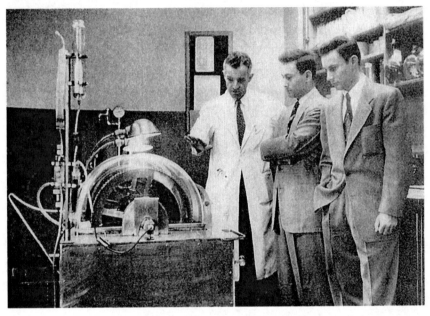

Dr. John Merrill discusses the artificial kidney with his patients, the Herrick Twins, in Boston after their successful surgery.

Chapter 9

Stanley Shaldon and his colleagues reported on their long term peritoneal dialysis program for chronic renal failure in April 1965. They concluded that if patients with chronic kidney failure and very low renal function didn't receive adequate dialysis time, they developed the "underdialysis syndrome." They believed these patients required at least 32 hours per week if they were to maintain positive health. *EDTA Proceedings; Vol. 2. Newcastle Upon Tyne; 1965 109-112.*

Chapter 10

W.G. Malette button procedure for peritoneal dialysis was used in 7 patients, from 3 days to over 20 months.with good results.

The Characteristics of Renal Hypoperfusion in Dogs with Acute and Chronic Reductions in Glomerular Filtration Rate as Disclosed by the Pattern of Water and Solute Excretion After Hypotonic Saline Infusions. George Van Giesen, Merrick Reese, Fredrik Kiil, Floyd Rector, Donald Seldin. *Journal of Clinical Investigation; Vol 43, 341 - 348*

The Mechanism of Salt Wastage in Chronic Renal Disease. Alan Coleman, Manuel Arias, Norman Carter, Floyd Rector, Donald Seldin. *Journal of Clinical Investigation, Vol 45, 116 - 125*

Other clinicians, *(Replacement of Renal Function by Dialysis, W. Drucker, Ed.,)* tried various plastic/Teflon conduits in a limited number of patients. None was successful for any significant period of time.

Chapter 11

The dietary management of patients with chronic progressive renal failure, in the early 1960s, before regular programs for dialysis were available, required very low protein (of high quality) intake. It was also necessary that patients were provided with sufficient calories—from fats, and especially vegetables and fruits—so as to not break down the patients' own body protein.

Many vegetables and fruits contain high levels of potassium, which needed to be restricted in these patients. Dieticians were very creative in fashioning diets following the G/G formulae for local/regional/national tastes. In our clinic, we found it useful to provide patients with a list of each food group arranged in a low potassium or high potassium column.

δ

The following is Christmas dinner menu typical of the low protein G/G diet for patients with severe chronic renal failure in the early 1960s in Edinburgh — modified for Scottish tastes:

> Turkey: as usual meat allowance for patient
>
> Stuffing: 0.5 oz. gluten free bread crumbs, 0.25 oz. suet, a pinch of mixed herbs, pepper — mix together and bind with a little water
>
> Cranberry sauce: 1 tsp.
>
> Bread sauce: 0.5 oz. gluten free bread from allowance, cream mixture (1 oz. cream and 2 oz. water). Simmer with onion, cloves, mace, and peppercorn. Remove onion, clove, and mace. Add bread crumbs and cook until thickened.
>
> Fruit salad: tinned
>
> Ice cream, meringue and cream with butter icing or brandy butter.

Web Site of the Edinburgh Renal Unit, Conservative treatment before dialysis was available, Chronic Renal Failure, Giovannetti Christmas Dinner, http://www.edren. org/pages/history/diet.php

Chapter 12

In the summer of 1944, Dr. Walter Kempner presented the results of his extensive research in patients with hypertensive vascular disease and kidney dysfunction at the annual meeting of the **American Medical Association in Chicago**. The talk was accompanied by detailed documentation of the effects of the "rice diet" in reversing heart failure, improving renal function, healing retinopathy, and lowering blood pressure in a significant number of patients.

Because of these dramatic changes attributed to the rice diet, some physicians and researchers accused Kempner of fraud, believing that he switched the dates on the before and after x rays of the heart and on the slides showing changes in the retina. Later, his results were fully validated by numerous unbiased clinical investigators and academicians.

A two volume set of Dr Kempner's scientific publications has been edited and published by Dr. Barbara Newborg, his chief medical associate for many years. Dr. Newborg has also written a book, **Walter Kempner and the Rice Diet**, about Kempner's life and times. A very readable, interesting, and informative narrative of a physician who challenged the conventional medical understanding of certain disease processes, and showed that previously "irreversible" conditions could, in fact, be reversed.

Chapter 13

Millard Smith M.D., working in Boston City Hospital, reported in the **Boston Medical and Surgical Journal (1927)** his experience in managing a teenage boy with chronic renal failure for 6 months on an extremely low (around 18 grams) protein diet. In 1963, Carmelo Giordano demonstrated the beneficial effects of a low (high biological value) protein diet on the clinical course of patients with chronic renal failure. Several years later, both Giordano and Sergio Giovannetti reported on a larger series of patients maintained on the G/G diet. Many of these patients were reported as being free of uremic symptoms for months to several years.

From Berlyne's experience in treating large numbers of patients with chronic renal failure with modifications of the G/G diet, it was apparent that, although uremic symptoms were drastically reduced in many patients, a new syndrome was emerging. Practically all symptoms related to the gastrointestinal tract were gone. Many patients did quite well untila few days before dying, when they became agitated. Some bled into their tissues, many developed acidosis and hyperkalemia. Death occurred quickly. *Berlyne et al. Proc. EDTA; Vol.2, 1965.*

Maintenance hemodialysis soon became the mainstay of therapy in chronic renal failure. Sergio Giovannetti, many years later (1989) pointed out "… clinical nephrologists were attracted by this therapy (maintenance hemodialysis) and interest in conservative therapy, including diet, declined or disappeared completely." *A Historical Rebiew of Low Protein Diets. Vol.7, Topics in Renal Medicine. S. Giovannetti*

Chapter 14

Belding Scribner, M.D., began giving regular hemodialysis treatments to a patient with chronic renal failure at the University of Washington in Seattle on March 9, 1960. On Scribner's team were Wayne Quinton, the hospital's biomedical engineer, and David Dillard, M.D. He and Scribner devised a shunt with Teflon tubing to be connected to the radial artery and an adjacent vein. Dillard, a pediatric cardiac surgeon, connected the shunt to the patient. The patient, Clyde Shields, a Boeing machinist, lived for 11 years on dialysis, dying from cardiac complications.

Scribner began dialyzing three additional patients later in the spring and early summer the same year, and wanted to expand the dialysis unit. The University of Washington was reluctant to expand. They were concerned that if Scribner's NIH funding dried up they would have to continue supporting dialysis patients.

Subsequently, Scribner obtained financial support from the Hartford Foundation. He moved his dialysis center from the hospital to the basement of the Swedish Hospital nurses residence. The Seattle Artificial Kidney Center opened there on January 1, 1962. *The Early History of Dialysis for Chronic Renal Failure in the United States: A View From Seattle. C.R. Blagg, M.D., 2007*

Chapter 15

Willem Kolff may have been the first to treat chronic renal failure with intestinal dialysis. In 1947, he dialyzed a uremic patient through an isolated ileal segment, improving the patient's condition enough that he was sent home to dialyze, with his wife performing the treatments. The patient lived for more than 60 days, eventually dying at home. *Oral Sorbents in Uremia, Eli Friedman; Replacement of Renal Function by Dialysis; Ed: Drucker, 1983*

Schloerb reported his experiences with intestinal dialysis in the *Journal of Clinical Investigation* in 1958. Over a period of 6-7 years, from the late 1950s until the early 1960s, he dialyzed 5 patients via the gastrointestinal tract. He recognized, early on, that complete restoration of renal function wasn't achievable with intestinal dialysis. However, during this period (late 1950s) he believed that this procedure "afforded uremic patients the best possibility for repeated dialysis to temporarily reduce uremic symptoms."

Chapter 16

Ethical considerations regarding the prolongation of patients' lives by artificial means were still a concern by physicians, in both academe and private practice. Irving Page, a prominent physician in research and clinical medicine, and editor of **Modern Medicine**, in 1963 wrote an editorial in which he referred to the experimental nature of dialysis, and the fact transplantations were not ready to be performed on a wide scale basis. In the same year, other academic physicians also were hesitant to recommend dialysis/transplantation as long-term therapies.

Robert Rettig, points out that is wasn't until 1967 that dialyzing patients with chronic renal failure received "official medical - scientific sanction." It was at that time that the **Gottschalk Committee**, set up by the government's Bureau of the Budget, gave its blessing to dialysis and transplantation as being safe and effective.

On a personal level, from the mid '60s, even through the early '70s, I frequently experienced questions from, especially, older friends and colleagues, whether it was "really a good idea" to keep chronic renal failure patients alive by dialyzing then on a regular basis.

Chapter 17

The "artificial kidney" that was purchased by the Women's Board of University Hospital was a model of the first commercially built "dialysis system," a result of the collaboration between Dr. Kolff and Dr. William Graham, CEO of Baxter Labs. The "system" was introduced in 1956, with a SigmaMotor (blood) pump and originally sold for $1200. The coil and blood lines sold for $59.

Later models substituted a roller type blood pump for the SigmaMotor pump, and commercially available dialysis solutions were added to the 100 liter tank and recirculated during the dialysis. The tank was emptied and fresh dialysate added every 2 hours. Even later, in the more efficient RSP model, dialysate entered a smaller container, was recirculated there before automatically being drained; thus not having to stop dialysing to empty the main tank. We purchased two used RSP models when we moved into our new dialysis center on 15th street.

Chapter 18

I had become very frustrated using peritoneal dialysis in trying to *properly* manage patients with chronic renal failure. Hemodialysis seemed to be out of the picture for the present. Yet, I had a number of patients with chronic renal failure in need of dialytic treatment. Opportunity would be closer than I anticipated.

Chapter 19

"After early efforts, the isolated intestinal loop procedure fell into disfavor because of inproved techniques for hemodialysis and the development of kidney transplantation and better methods of kidney harvesting and immune suppression. *Paul Schloerb; ASAIO Trans. 36: 4 – 7 1990*

Chapter 20

Arthur Humphries as head of the transplantation team at the **Medical College of Georgia** was attentive to every detail of his patients' condition, both in the surgery suite as well as in the pre and post transplant days. This characteristic served him and his patients well, as reflected in the success of MCG's kidney transplant program over the years.

Chapter 21

In an article in the **Los Angeles Times, August 1991**, by Pamela Warrick, John Darrah recalls receiving a letter from The Seattle Artificial Kidney Centers Admission and Policies

Committee requesting that he serve on their committee. Darrah, a retired minister of Magnolia Lutheran Church in Seattle, said his first reaction was "No thank you." He did attend their first meeting where one of the "kidney doctors" explained that committee members were not being asked to decide who's going to die. That had already been determined. The doctor told them that most of the patients would die within several weeks. They were being asked to decide who would be given an opportunity to live. Darrah agreed to be on the committee, and served for nine years as the chairman of that committee, until he moved to California.

Chapter 22

In 1966, the *NEJM* reported that the AV fistula, which revolutionized the approach to hemodialysis, was created by the team of Brescia, Cimino, Appel, and Hurwich at the VA Hospital, Bronx, New York,. Twelve of the first 14 AV fistulas functioned without complications and 2 failed completely. Dr Scribner is reported to have been the first physician to refer one of his patients to New York for the creation of an AV fistula. **Nephrology Dialysis, Transplant, Dec 2005**

Chapter 23

"In 1955, I went to the Chairman of the Department of Research (Cleveland Clinic). That was Dr. Irving Page — a great scientist — but not particularly interested in artificial kidneys. I said, 'Dr. Page, will you give me three weeks because I think I can make a disposable artificial kidney.' He gave me three weeks and in that time, with the help of Wachener, who came from Austria to work with us, we made the twin coil artificial kidney. The twin coil artificial kidney made dialysis possible worldwide. The twin coil artificial kidney consists of window screening, the screening that you use to keep the flies out of your house, wound around a fruit juice can and then between the bindings there is the artificial sausage skin — the cellophane tubing. When I bought the various parts of it in a hardware store, the total cost was $16.25 and Baxter Laboratories, to which we gave the twin coil artificial kidney, sold them for $62. But they did succeed in making dialysis worldwide and they paid for it in the beginning and they built their entire artificial organ division on that twin coil artificial kidney. That was Baxter Laboratories. The Division that did it was Travenol." *ISN Video Legacy Project; University of Utah. Interview of Dr. Willem Kolff by David Ahlstrom, Oct. 27, 1995*

Chapter 24

In 1966, at the annual meeting of the *American Society of Artificial Internal Organs*, in Atlantic City, Donald Snyder and John Merrill presented their experience with sauna baths as a "therapeutic tool" in the treatment of chronic uremia. They enrolled 8 patients to take sauna baths on the days they were not dialyzed. A significant amount of fluid was removed via the sauna treatments to allow a liberalization of fluid intake in the patients' dietary regimen. Added benefits included relief from uremic pruritis, eliminating "urea and other end products of metabolism," modest reductions in blood pressure, and an overall improved "sense of well being."

Chapter 25

From the early 1960s until the 1972 statute *(Public Law 92-603)* covering essentially all patients with chronic kidney failure, each dialysis center had its own criteria for accepting patients into their programs. Many had committees similar to the Seattle Artificial Kidney Center. Others were more liberal about patients' ages and about specific diseases. Very few accepted diabetics. When the 1972 law was passed some of the burden of decision making was removed from the committees and the physician nephrologists—at least from the financial aspect.

Latest data from the **US Renal Data System (March 31, 2015)** show almost 700,000 patients being dialyzed in the US. Over a third of these patients are diabetics. Estimates suggest that the total worldwide number of dialysis patients is over 2 million.

Chapter 26

General Mills launched their coupon redemption promotion in 1929. In 1969, the Kidney Foundation of Ohio (KFO) wrote General Mills asking if they would approve KFO holding a coupon drive to purchase an artificial kidney, 600,000 coupons were to be redeemed for a $3000 "kidney." Under the Betty Crocker name, General Mills approved the program. More than 300 dialysis machines were purchased by other organizations—state kidney foundations and other medical groups.

Almost as soon as these programs began, bad publicity caused General Mills to rescind them. Some characterized the company as trading in human misery. In December 1970, they discontinued the program. *Manufacturing Tales: Sex and Money in Contemporary Legends; Gary A. Fine 1992.*

Chapter 27

When Hy Sussman joined me in practice, I had already moved from Harper Street to a larger office on 15th Street, across from MCG's Talmadge Hospital. From a one-chair dialysis clinic to a 3-station center. Our home training programs were fully functioning.

Chapter 28

Home hemodialysis. began in the early 1960s in Seattle (Scribner), Boston (Merrill), and London (Shaldon). Shaldon soon began dialyzing overnight, after having designed procedures and equipment to ensure safety and efficiency. Overenight Hemodialysis in the Home. *Proc. EDTA; Vol. 2 1965*

Chapter 29

"The instruction manual for the artificial kidney reveals that the seemingly simple concept of diffusion is not so easily carried out. Operation of the Travenol RSP required a large amount of preparation and continuous monitoring and attention for it to safely cleanse a patient's blood." *Case Western Reserve University, College of Arts and Sciences, Dittrick Medical History Center. "Comments about Travenol Artificial Kidney; Circa 1963." http://artsci.case.edu/dittrick/online-exhibits/explore-the-artifacts/artificial-kidney-1963/ (last updated November 14, 2014).*

Chapter 30

In a 1968 article in the *Transactions of the American Society for Artificial Organs,* Ornesti stated that the place for bilateral nephrectomy in patients with chronic renal failure was not definitively agreed upon. But, he suggested that there were three conditions in which it should be performed:

1. dialysis patients with uncontrolled hypertension (resistant to drugs and sodium depletions)
2. patients who cannot/will not stay on their low salt diets
3. most patients with malignant hypertension. ***

Budisavljevic, commenting on Calciphylaxis in chronic renal failure, in the *Journal of the American Society of Nephrology, July 1996*, pointed out that the lack of understanding of the cause of the condition makes treating it unsatisfactory. He notes further that some patients do improve following removal of the parathyroid glands but the prognosis for the disease is poor and mortality high.

As late as 2016, the mortality rate in calciphylaxis patients was near 70% as reported by Ozdemir's group in the *Casplan J of Internal Medicine*. They state, "early parathyroidectomy may be lifesaving."

Chapter 31

Today, *Center* hemodialysis remains a highly technical and intricate procedure. Over the years, repeated efforts have been made to encourage *Home* dialysis, for which there are many advantages: setting your own dialysis times, feeling more in control of your life, being better able to keep your job, generally feeling better and "enjoying life" more, and having less frequent clinic visits, to mention a few.

However, incentives for home dialysis training are lacking. Patients often report not knowing they even have a choice. Dialysis physicians (and dialysis clinics) frequently don't have the setup for training and follow-up for Home dialysis. Moreover, the financial inducements for physicians and patients are inadequate.

In recent years, some in the dialysis community have been devising "systems" for home hemodialysis that may help fill this void. Baxter recently announced an "investigational home dialysis system, Vivia, that includes an integrated water purification module, safety sensors, and one button fluid infusion." This system also includes a "two-way connectivity platform that allows physicians and nurses to monitor patients' treatment results remotely." *Business Wire website, Baxter Enrolls First Patient in U.S. Clinical Trial for VIVIA Investigational Home Hemodialysis System, March 15, 2016, http://www.businesswire.com/news/home/20160315005870/ en/Baxter-Enrolls-Patient-U.S.-Clinical-Trial-VIVIA; Also Baxter website, Baxter Enrolls First Patient in U.S. Clinical Trial for VIVIA Investigational Home Hemodialysis System, March 15, 2016, http://www.baxter.com/news-media/*

newsroom/press-releases/2016/03-15-16-vivian-clin3-trial-release.page

An even more interesting and (?) less costly system, Tablo, marketed by Outset Medical, is presently undergoing clinical trials. According to the company's web site, the machine was designed for "ease of patients' use." It's compact, about 35 inches in height, uses plain tap water to create the dialysing solution, monitors blood pressure, and delivers medications. It's described as a "consumer product with a touchscreen and 3-D animation and instructions." *Fierce Medical Devices Website, Outset Medical rounds up $91M to make dialysis options more attractive, June 8, 2015, http://www.fiercebiotech.com/medical-devices/outset-medical-rounds-up-91m-to-make-dialysis-options-more-attractive*

ABOUT THE AUTHOR

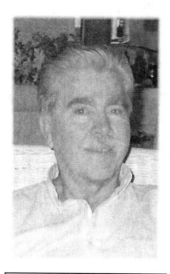 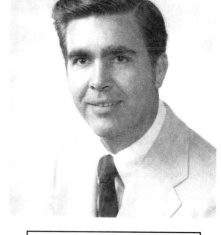

Dr. Van Giesen today   **Dr. Van Giesen in 1971**

GEORGE VAN GIESEN received his M.D. from the Medical College of Georgia (MCG). Following his Internship, Medical Residency, and Nephrology Fellowship at University of Texas Southwestern Medical School in Dallas, he began practicing medicine in Augusta, Georgia.

Serving on the clinical faculty at MCG, he established the chronic dialysis program at Talmadge Hospital, MCG's main teaching facility. He founded The Augusta Dialysis Center. the first outpatient dialysis facility in the Central Savannah River Area (CSRA). He was closely involved with the establishment of the Garden City Rescue Mission and the planning and construction of Doctors Hospital in west Augusta.

After his retirement he moved back to his hometown, Savannah, Georgia where he lives on the Moon River with his wife, Sylvia.